SUPPORT FOR THE AND THE DYING IN SERVICES FOR ADULTS WITH AUTISTIC SPECTRUM DISORDERS

A guide for managers and service staff

Helen Green Allison

First published 2001 by The National Autistic Society, 393 City Road, London EC1V 1NG

All rights reserved. No part of this publication may be reproduced, stored in a retrieval system or transmitted, in any form or by any means, electronic, mechanical, photocopying, recording or otherwise without the prior permission of the copyright owner.

ISBN 1 899 280 66 9

© The National Autistic Society

Designed and typeset by Column Communications

Printed in Great Britain by Crowes

Acknowledgements

Sincere thanks are owed to all those who gave valuable help and support during the preparation of this revised work. They are as follows:

- **David Potter**, Information Centre Manager, The National Autistic Society, who has been immensely helpful in identifying and searching out references, supervising the process, and answering questions promptly, always with unfailing patience and courtesy.

- **Norman Green**, Company Secretary, The National Autistic Society, who advised on copyright issues.

- **Fred Parsons**, Director, Nottingham Regional Society for Autistic Children and Adults, who read through the draft and contributed the important sections relating to sudden death in services.

- **Silu Pascoe**, Inspector, Social Services Inspectorate, who not only read through the draft, but spent hours proofreading it, identifying errors which had escaped my notice and suggesting helpful amendments.

- **Mick Taylor**, House Manager, Somerset Court, who read the draft and offered encouragement and helpful suggestions.

The help of those who were kind enough to contribute their experiences of supporting bereaved people with autism have been acknowledged in the introduction to the Appendices. Particular mention has been made of the valuable contribution by the young man with Asperger syndrome who described his own experiences of bereavement.

Preface

My paper, *The Management of Bereavement in Services for People with Autism,* was written in 1992 with advice from managers of services for adults with autism. The introduction to that paper was as follows:

"Until recently, people with learning disabilities have been denied the right to grieve, on the mistaken assumption that they had no capacity to do so. This process of dehumanisation has been made all the more poignant by the movement towards advocating their rights in other areas (Kitching, 1987). Recognition both of their right and their capacity to grieve has led to a realisation that staff caring for people with learning disabilities should be trained to enable them, when they suffer loss, to complete the tasks of grieving in their own way and in their own time."

I hope that the right of people with autistic spectrum disorders not only to grieve but to be offered appropriate support in their grieving is now accepted in all services caring for them. However, I have revised my original work because of the impact of ageing on those cared for in services for adults: there is recognition of a greater need for preparation for bereavement management and the introduction of preparation for care of the dying. Increasing numbers of people with Asperger syndrome are now being diagnosed and terminology has also changed.

Much of the information regarding preparation for bereavement as well as strategies for support is still valid for the management of bereavement in children.

Appendix I 'Grief reactions of people with autism' was compiled from the results of a survey undertaken as the basis for the original paper. It is no less valid at present than it was in 1992. Only one of those included was described as having Asperger syndrome, but it is likely that some of the others would now be similarly diagnosed.

Appendix II 'Grief reactions of people with Asperger syndrome' was compiled from the results of a request for those who supported people with Asperger syndrome to supply information for the present paper, similar to that in the first survey. Very few responses were received. However, I am grateful to those who did respond and to the young man with Asperger syndrome who offered a very moving analysis of his bereavement experience.

Contents

Purpose of this book	9
Part I Bereavement management: the need for preparation	11
Introduction	11
Responses to bereavement	12
The process of grieving	13
Factors affecting responses to grief	14
Relating responses to grief to those on the autistic spectrum	15
Types of bereavement	15
Ageing parents – ways for helping them maintain family contact	16
Part II Preparation for bereavement management	17
Preparation is the key: objectives and strategies	17
Forming a bereavement support group	18
Bereavement questionnaire	18
Encouraging parents to consider their own funeral arrangements so that their son or daughter can participate	19
Encouraging parents to make provision for the welfare of their son or daughter after their own deaths	20
Parents' wishes in respect of the death of their family member	22

Practical arrangements following the death of a service user 22

Preparing staff to manage bereavement 24

Understanding individual clients 25

Training staff to provide loss and death education for service users 27

Preparing people with autism for loss and bereavement 27

Training staff to support clients when bereavement occurs 31

Part III Supportive measures for bereaved people with autism 33

Designating members of staff to support bereaved clients 33

Anticipated or sudden death: informing the client 34

Initiating bereavement management 35

Comforting the bereaved 42

Facilitating access to therapeutic measures 43

Facilitating supportive relationships 44

Coping with grief reactions 44

Absence of grief following bereavement 48

Problems encountered in bereavement of people with autism 48

Anniversaries 53

Part IV Other aspects of bereavement support — 55

Support of surviving family members — 55

Support of staff caring for a bereaved client — 55

Loss of client or loss of staff member — 56

Part V Support for the dying — 59

Care of the dying — 59

Training for support staff — 59

Needs of support staff — 60

Knowing the individual patient well — 60

Communication: the need for tranquillity and a consistent approach — 60

Communication with the patient: the need for tact and care — 61

The religious dimension — 62

The patient's physical comfort — 62

Appropriate diet — 62

Location — 63

Access to palliative care — 63

Issues relating to palliative care for people with learning disabilities — 64

Commitment to the dying — 65

Appendices Grief reactions of people with autistic spectrum disorders 67

Appendix I Grief reactions of people with autism 69

Appendix II Grief reactions of people with Asperger syndrome 89

References: Bereavement 95

Support for the dying 99

Useful addresses 101

Index 107

The purpose of this book

The main purpose of this book is to offer guidelines so that staff in services for people with autism can offer confident, informed and sensitive support to those in their care in the event of bereavement.

There is a great deal of easily accessible literature on bereavement, and it is strongly recommended that staff familiarise themselves with the common responses to bereavement by referring to it (see Part I, References and Useful Addresses). This book will draw attention to the responses to bereavement of people with autistic spectrum disorders, and will suggest ways in which staff can train themselves in the management of bereavement, both in its practical aspects and in offering support to clients, staff and others who might be affected by bereavement occurring in services for people with autism.

It cannot be overemphasised that because of the individual nature of reactions to bereavement and the grieving process, this book cannot be prescriptive. I can only suggest measures which can be adapted to individuals or from which a choice can be made.

Because support for the dying will become increasingly important in services for people with autism it is hoped that some of the suggestions made in Part V may be helpful to staff who undertake this very demanding role.

PART I

Bereavement management: the need for preparation

> "There is no growth without
> pain and conflict and no loss
> that cannot lead to gain"
> *(Pincus, 1961)*

Introduction

The process of ageing is becoming ever more relevant to services caring for adults with autistic spectrum disorders. It follows that awareness of the issues surrounding bereavement – loss and death – is becoming an increasingly important component of the caring role as deaths of parents, of service staff and of service users themselves become more frequent. Accordingly, the need for staff to prepare themselves to offer effective practical and emotional support for service users through bereavement and death has become a matter of urgency.

The term 'autism' in this book is used to refer to autistic spectrum disorders. The main criteria for diagnosis of these disorders is the following triad of impairments: social interaction, social communication and imagination (inflexibility of thought), accompanied by repetitive behaviour patterns and resistance to change. The spectrum includes a wide range of cognitive disabilities, from severe intellectual disability to average or above average intelligence (The National Autistic Society, 1998). The paper *How many people have autistic spectrum disorders?* (1997), obtainable from The National Autistic Society, offers a brief but comprehensive analysis of autistic spectrum disorders.

Throughout this book the term 'services' applies not only to residential and day care establishments, but also to outreach services supporting people with autism living independently in the community. In the interests of brevity, the term 'client' is used to designate 'service user.' The word 'parent' is used to refer to any person who fulfils the parental role in relation to the service user including, for example, a significant family member or friend if there is no living or interested parent.

Responses to bereavement

Bereavement can be defined as 'the loss of something that is precious' (Pincus, 1996). It usually refers to the death of someone close, but can include a significant change in one's life or the loss of a significant object. All of these life events may evoke a grieving process in clients, and staff should be aware of this. The most catastrophic loss, however, is usually brought about by the death of a person.

Studies of people with learning disabilities have shown that of those who for no apparent reason suddenly presented with emotional and management difficulties, approximately half had experienced the death or loss of someone close prior to the onset of symptoms (Emerson, 1977). Similar results were shown in a study of admissions to an acute psychiatric ward of people with learning disabilities suffering from neurosis (Day, 1985). A limited cognitive capacity does not indicate a limited emotional capacity (Sireling, quoted in Kitchling, 1987).

Whether or not they are learning disabled, people react individually to grief, but most people share certain reactions. Because people with autism are impaired in their social interactions, it might be concluded that they do not form attachments to other people and are therefore insulated from the grieving process. Statements have been made by individuals, one high functioning autistic (Schneider, 1999) and one with Asperger syndrome (Gillberg, 1991), which appear to confirm this. However, surveys undertaken of those who have supported people with autism through the grieving process have indicated that many have been deeply affected by the death of someone close (Appendix II and Rawlings, 1998).

The examples available of people with autism who have successfully coped with grief are those who have received skilled support either from family members or members of staff. On the basis of such evidence, five further conclusions can be reached:
- All people with autism react individually to bereavement and the approach to support, if required, needs to be as unique as the individual involved.
- They may share the common responses to bereavement and may be affected by the major determinants of reactions to grief.
- The grieving processes of people with autism are profoundly affected by their disabilities
- They may undergo reactions similar to those of bereaved children and young people.
- The problems and reactions of bereaved people with other learning disabilities may also be experienced by people with autism.

It follows that training resources and publications relating to bereavement in children and people with learning disabilities can be helpful to those caring for people with autism.

The process of grieving

Any or all of these responses to grief may be experienced by bereaved people. Many experts view grief as a process with identifiable stages:
- shock, numbness, denial
- despair, turmoil and acute grieving, including:
  - anger
  - guilt
  - anxiety, fear, panic
  - depression
  - pain, appetite disturbance, breathlessness, illness
  - more than usual need for sleep, sleeplessness, hyperactivity
  - nightmares
  - regression, loss of skills.
- recovery
  - acceptance
  - resolution of grief
  - when the bereaved can think of the deceased without pain or anger and can recall the times they had together in a positive way.

These concepts are helpful, provided it is understood that people do not experience an orderly progression from one stage to the other. These stages are responses which may overlap and merge with each other (Carr, 1988). The shock/denial stage may last for hours or weeks. The other stages last longer and have no time limit. Normally, mourning the loss of a close relationship takes a year and may take as long as two years (Worden, 1991).

Acceptance and recovery do not imply that the grief is over. It can be felt throughout life, sometimes as a stab of pain, but also in the form of a memory of shared experience. Anniversaries are particularly difficult, for example, the date of the death, of birthdays, the celebration of Christmas and other festivals which might have been shared with the deceased.

Unresolved or complicated grief occurs when the bereaved has failed fully to

experience the stages of grief or to have performed the tasks of mourning identified by J. Worden (1991):
- accepting the reality of loss
- experiencing the pain of grief
- adjusting to an environment in which the deceased is missing
- emotionally relocating the deceased and to move on with life.

Factors affecting the responses to grief (based on Worden (1991))

The intensity and duration of responses to grief common to all people suffering from bereavement are affected by a combination of important factors. Who the deceased was and the closeness of the relationship to the bereaved is of great importance. The nature of the attachment, its strength and security, or the ambivalence of the relationship, including any conflicts during the lifetime of the deceased, may influence the reaction.

The mode of death – whether it occurred suddenly or with advance warning – has an impact, too. It is usually easier to accept the death of a person ripe in years than that of a young person. Natural deaths are more easily accepted than accidental deaths; suicides and homicides are particularly hard to accept. Another dimension associated with the mode of death is where it occurred geographically, whether nearby or far away.

Historical factors also play a part. The bereaved person's previous experiences of grieving, for example, the irresolution of a previous death, may affect reactions to a subsequent one. Those with a history of depression will have difficulty in coping with bereavement.

The personality, age and sex of the bereaved will also influence their response. So, too, will their ability to handle anxiety and stress, whether they have difficulty in expressing themselves and whether they are highly dependent or if they have problems forming relationships. People diagnosed with certain personality disorders may find it difficult to handle loss.

Social variables are significant, too. Ethnic and religious backgrounds, including grieving rituals, as well as the degree of perceived emotional and social support from others, influence the responses of the bereaved. Their lives may be further affected during the grieving process by other stressful, disruptive and possibly life-changing events following the death.

Relating responses to grief to those on the autistic spectrum

Staff wishing to offer support to a bereaved client need to bear in mind the major factors determining responses to grief when briefing themselves about the individual concerned. They also need to be aware of the ways that autism and the client's position on the spectrum can affect their grieving process. These factors will be discussed in various contexts in this book, but it should be pointed out here that the wide variation in the capabilities of people with autism introduces an additional complexity into the functions of staff offering support to bereaved clients. For example, a client at the able end of the spectrum may require detailed explanations and opportunities to explore their own concepts of death and after-life beliefs. Those in the mid-range of the autistic spectrum would probably derive most comfort from simple, factual, directive language. Those at the more disabled end of the spectrum might be confused by any but the minimum of information. Staff must be prepared, therefore, to respond with flexibility, depending on the ability of the bereaved individual.

Specific grief reactions of people with autism are described in the Appendices. It is important to bear these in mind as they may help staff to interpret the reactions of those in their care.

Types of bereavement

Bereavement in services for people with autism may take a variety of forms. It may involve losses other than death of someone close affecting the individual client, such as moving the family home, the break-up of parents' marriage or siblings moving from family home. The transfer from one living environment to another and staff changes, the loss of a pet or loss of precious possession may have a profound impact on their lives, too.

It may, however, involve the loss of a family member or someone close to the individual client. The loss of a second parent is particularly difficult to accept because of the fundamental life changes which may follow. The death of a fellow service user or a staff member may affect a client, too.

The greater part of this book is concerned with the loss of a family member, but most of the suggestions made in this context can apply to the death of a fellow service user or a staff member. These are discussed more briefly but they can have a profound impact on the survivors within the services.

Ageing parents: ways of helping them maintain family contact

Before giving details of the preparations for bereavement management itself, it is important to outline the problems faced by ageing parents and the ways in which services caring for their son or daughter can help both client and parent maintain their relationship.

Safeguards for the lone parent

As clients age it becomes more likely, either because of death or divorce, that they are left with only one parent, who will be their sole carer during home visits. This poses the risk that should the parent become seriously ill or incapacitated the client will be left alone, lacking the ability to call for help. Accordingly, staff in the service should ensure that someone suitable is found to live with the parent during the client's home visits. Should this not be possible, staff need to advise the parent that they should make an agreement with a staff member or with a reliable friend or relative to telephone them at an agreed time every day, or, alternatively, that they themselves should undertake to telephone someone daily at an agreed time. If contact is not made, the staff, relative or friend can immediately take whatever action is necessary.

Supporting parents in a changing situation

As parents age they will inevitably have diminished stamina, and because of the disabilities which accompany old age, they may find that they are unable to continue to provide the home visits which had become an important part of the lives of both themselves and of their son or daughter. Ending home visits by the client at Christmas, Easter and birthdays can be traumatic for both parties. Parents may find it difficult or impossible either to drive or to travel on public transport to visit the service premises.

This problem should not be allowed to erode the family relationship, bearing in mind that meaningful telephone conversation with a person with autism may not be an option. Staff can take an active role in preserving the relationship by enabling client visits to their parents in their own home with staff support, taking them on outings together, or making arrangements for the parents' visits to the service. Staff can also help by booking local overnight accommodation for parents living some distance away. Alternatively, services, where possible, can provide guest accommodation for parents on the premises.

PART II

Preparation for bereavement management

Preparation is the key

Preparation for the management of bereavement services for people with autism should have clear objectives. Putting in place a sound set of procedures, working in co-operation with the client's family where possible and sensitive staff training are all essential components of this planning process.

Strategies to support the client and involve his or her family
- Ensure that relevant information about service users is readily available in the event of bereavement or death. This should include details of the client's previous losses, ethnic and religious background, contact details of significant persons and forms of address used by service users for those close to them.
- Encourage parents to plan the rituals surrounding their own deaths so that they may be meaningful for their family member, and to inform staff of measures which will help to comfort when bereavement occurs.
- Encourage parents to plan for the welfare of their son or daughter after their own death, in particular by financial planning and provision of supportive relationships.
- Invite parents to record their wishes in respect of the death of their family member and, if possible, to plan accordingly to ensure that funds are available for the funeral and burial or cremation arrangements.
- Be prepared to undertake the practical arrangements necessary following the death of a service user.
- Be prepared to offer help to surviving family members in understanding, or at least coming to terms with, the reactions of bereaved clients.
- Be prepared to offer support to surviving family members in the event of the death of a client.
- Ensure that bereaved clients are supported during this time by designated members of staff who know them well and who understand the grieving process.
- Facilitate other supportive relationships for bereaved clients.

Training measures for service staff to help their bereaved clients
- Make sure that staff have the background knowledge for bereavement management in this context: a sound understanding of autism and of individual clients, their personalities and significant facts about them; knowing how to make appropriate funeral arrangements and how to approach and support relatives.
- Train staff to provide education about loss and death for clients to enable them to cope with bereavement when the time comes.
- Train staff to help clients when bereavement occurs, for example, making the rituals of death more meaningful to their clients, supporting them in their own ways of grieving, and in forming concepts of death and after-life beliefs.
- Ensure that staff receive the support they need in the management of a client's bereavement, when caring for a client facing death, and when coping with their own grief in the event of the death of clients or colleagues.

Ways of meeting these objectives are proposed on the understanding that each bereavement is unique and that staff responsible for the management of bereavement will need to decide which measures are appropriate in any particular circumstance.

Forming a bereavement support group

The formation of bereavement support groups within services is one of the recommended ways of helping to implement successful bereavement management, to monitor it, and to ensure that standards of bereavement training are appropriately met.

Membership of a bereavement support group could include members of staff of the service who have received bereavement training, members of the local clergy and other representatives from the religions of service users. Members of CRUSE, The Compassionate Friends, the Samaritans (see Useful Addresses) and relatives of service users are also invaluable contributors to such a group.

Bereavement questionnaire

Collecting relevant information about clients, while also encouraging parents to make arrangements for the future of their family member after their own death will considerably ease bereavement management. A bereavement questionnaire

should include the following sections.
a) Factual information which will enable staff to offer effective support to an individual bereaved client, including previous losses, how the parents wish him or her to be informed of their death, where advice should be sought to help participation in the rituals surrounding death and the forms of address used for people close to the client.
b) Financial provision for the client by way of a Will or Settlement and how it can be accessed on their behalf by the service caring for them.
c) The names and contact details of people who have been nominated to perform some functions previously provided by the deceased parent, such as home visits, friendship, advocacy.
d) Parents' wishes in respect of arrangements following the death of their family member.
e) Family members' own views on death (if these have been expressed).

A sample questionnaire, which can be adapted for use for adults, is available from The National Autistic Society and archived on the NAS website (see Useful Addresses). Although it is desirable that the questionnaire be completed by parents on admission of their family member to the service, they may wish to do this in stages as their plans for the future develop. The completed questionnaire should be kept in a confidential file and the service should ensure that it is periodically reviewed, possibly at the client's annual review meeting, so that it can be updated as necessary.

Encouraging parents to consider their own funeral arrangements so that their family member can participate

If their relationship with the client's parents allows them to do so, staff may wish to encourage them to consider how their own funeral arrangements and burial or cremation rituals might be made meaningful for their son or daughter with autism. Clients then may be able to participate. Staff should make themselves available to discuss with parents how this might be achieved, perhaps when they are completing the bereavement questionnaire.

Parents should, in any case, inform staff of their wishes in this regard, either through the bereavement questionnaire or by means of a letter to be attached to the client's file.

Staff may need to remind parents, particularly those who wish their remains to be cremated, that some people with autism need a focus for their grieving process in the form of a memorial stone which they can visit and where they can plant a rose bush or lay flowers.

Encouraging parents to make provision for the welfare of their son or daughter after their own deaths

If communication between staff and parents is well established, staff will be in a position to encourage parents to prepare for the future welfare of their family member with autism after their own deaths. This preparation includes financial provision by way of Settlement or Will and provision of supportive relationships for their family member in the event of death or incapacity of both parents.

The arrangements made should be recorded in the bereavement questionnaire so that there is a permanent record accessible to staff at the time of the parents' death.

Financial provision by way of Settlement or Will

Before making any financial arrangement by way of Settlement or Will in order to benefit their son or daughter, parents are strongly advised to obtain the document *Financial provision by way of Settlement or Will for people with autism* from The National Autistic Society. This gives advice on briefing a solicitor so that any provision made will not threaten entitlement to government or local authority funding.

The bereavement questionnaire invites parents to record any such arrangements and how the service can obtain access to the benefit for the client. This would mean that after the parents' deaths, the service is able to call upon funds to provide something special for the client, such as a piece of equipment or a holiday.

Provision of supportive relationships in the event of death or incapacity of both parents

These supportive relationships can take the form either of a 'successor parent' who takes over the parents' caring and advocacy roles, or a 'citizen advocate' who, strictly speaking, serves as an advocate for the client but may also serve in the caring role. Both functions, in order to be effective, must be undertaken by people considerably closer in age to the client than the parents. It is helpful to all concerned – clients, parents and staff – if they have been selected by the parents while they are able still to take an active part in briefing them for their role and in familiarising them with the aims of the service caring for the client.

Successor parent

The 'successor parent' is usually either a sibling of the client, a relative or a family friend, but they should have expressed a clear wish to serve in this capacity. Whether or not siblings have been chosen as successor parents, staff will wish to build up a relationship between them and the service caring for the family member with autism. However, this needs to be undertaken with sensitivity as some siblings may not wish to be involved. The term successor parent is used in preference to 'befriender' because the former implies a long-term commitment to undertake aspects of the parental role. This in no way denigrates the role of befriender which can help to enrich the life of a person with autism by providing companionship.

Citizen advocate (see Useful Addresses)

The appointment of a 'citizen advocate' may have a more formal dimension than that of the successor parent, although the advocate may serve in this capacity as well. In some cases, staff may consider it wise to reinforce their clients' access to effective advocacy by appointing citizen advocates for them, preferably in co-operation with their parents. A citizen advocate is an individual (usually non-disabled) who advocates for the client, representing their interests as though they were their own. So that there may be no conflict of interests, a citizen advocate should be independent of any service directly affecting the client, and they should have no familial connections with them.

Staff, with the consent of parents, may need to take an active part in the selection and appointment of citizen advocates because they may be more likely to have access to groups able to provide for them. As soon as a citizen advocate is appointed, they will have a standing in relation to the client which must be recognised by the service caring for them. A conscientious citizen advocate will wish to get to know the client well so that he or she can represent them effectively.

Building relationships between the successor parent, citizen advocate and the client

During the lifetime of the parent and in co-operation with them, service staff should take measures to facilitate these supportive relationships for the client. Their aim should be to work for a seamless transfer of the caring and advocacy roles in the event of the incapacity or death of the parent.

Staff can welcome visits to the client by the successor parent and/or citizen advocate and make them feel free to discuss in private the client's personality and interests by telephone or during visits to the service. It is also important to keep them informed of the client's activities. Another valuable strategy is to invite them to attend the client's annual review meetings, parent partnership meetings and any other discussions of the client's progress and future development.

It is also very helpful to include their names on mailing lists for the in-house news magazine and any important notices.

Parents' wishes in respect of the death of their family member

A bereavement questionnaire can invite parents to record their wishes in respect of the death of their family member. The National Autistic Society's service policy is to encourage relatives to consider funding funeral plans which will cover all eventualities during or after their lifetime. Where no arrangements are in place, The National Autistic Society undertakes to meet the cost of a dignified funeral which reflects the cultural, religious or other aspects of the individual.

It is clearly beneficial if parents ensure that the necessary funds are available for the funeral and burial or cremation of their family member. This relieves the service of the considerable financial pressures which can accrue as a result of caring for an ageing group of clients.

Parents will wish to consider whether they prefer to make these funds available by means of a pre-paid funeral plan or by a Will or Settlement. Advice on the former can be obtained through local undertaking firms. In any event, the service must do its best to fulfil the parents' stated wishes concerning the type of funeral service (religious denomination, secular or humanist), burial or cremation arrangements and preferred type of memorial.

If parents are still living when their family member dies and they or other relatives want to be involved in funeral arrangements, it is hoped that they will reach an agreement with staff on how the responsibility will be shared.

Practical arrangements following the death of a service user

Services caring for adults with autism must be prepared to take responsibility for the practical arrangements for notification and registration of the death of a service user, as well as facilitating the funeral and cremation or burial. If the doctors deems it necessary to report the death to the coroner, there may be a post mortem examination of the body and possibly an inquest. Staff members who are willing to take responsibility for these necessary procedures at short notice should read and keep for reference *What to do when someone dies* (Harris, 1998) (see References) and the most recent edition of *What to do after a death in England and Wales,* obtainable free of charge from the local Benefits Agency. Information booklets may be available from local undertakers and from the local cemetery and crematorium.

Religious and ethnic background of the deceased

When a client dies and before the staff initiate any action regarding the laying out of the body and the rituals surrounding death, close regard must be paid to the religious and ethnic background of the deceased. Different religions have their own practices regarding the preparation of the body and its burial or cremation.

If links have not already been made as a result of their clients' regular attendance at a place of worship, it is important that, as a preparatory measure, staff find out how to contact religious and other relevant groups so that the rituals surrounding their deaths are appropriate to their religious and ethnic backgrounds.

Taking primary responsibility for the client's funeral arrangements

In the event that the service may have to take the primary responsibility for the funeral arrangements of a service user, it may be wise for staff to get in touch with several local undertakers so that they may brief themselves on what is involved and the options which are available. They should be aware that undertaking is a business and that efforts are made to sell as many services as possible.

When arranging a funeral, it is important to obtain at least two estimates and compare costs. There can be a great deal of flexibility in funeral arrangements, and it is possible to organise a simple, dignified and relatively inexpensive funeral in which mourners can take an active part.

CRUSE advises that it is a good training strategy for staff to visit an undertaker (making it clear that it is a training exercise) to negotiate the type of funeral that they would like to have for themselves. It also suggests that those responsible for funeral negotiations be prepared to ask someone not directly involved to accompany them, to give an objective view and to support them in requesting some time to think about the options before making decisions. Staff may also find it helpful to attend an open day at a crematorium so that they will know what to expect if they have to arrange a cremation.

Getting to know the vicar, priest or other religious leader in the local community

If it is possible to establish a link with the vicar, priest or other religious leader locally, s/he can be a valuable source of advice when making arrangements for a funeral, burial, cremation or memorial service, as well as helping with the support of bereaved clients or staff. The link may already have been made by clients' regular attendance at local religious services and, if willing, then the religious representative can become a valuable member of the bereavement support group, and perhaps help with staff training for bereavement management.

Preparing staff to manage bereavement: ground rules

It is essential that staff supporting people with autism through the grieving process should not only understand the common responses to bereavement, but they should also have an understanding of autism and of the individual personality, the previous losses and the relationships of the person to whom they are offering support, and any other significant facts. This will enable them not only to interpret the reactions of the bereaved but also to provide support in ways which can circumvent the barriers of their disabilities, the triad of impairments and associated conditions. This knowledge will help make staff training in bereavement effective.

Training in bereavement management should enable staff to provide education about loss and death for service users in preparation for bereavement and enable them to support service users when bereavement occurs.

Knowledge of autism and communication strategies

So that staff are aware how autism and the client's position on the spectrum can affect their grieving process, the service needs to give staff access to suitable training courses and make literature on autism available in the service library. There is, however, no substitute for 'hands on' experience.

Staff training should promote an understanding of the use of non-verbal communication with people with autism such as signing, and the use of signs, symbols and photographs, all of which can be usefully combined with each other as well as with verbal communication (The National Autistic Society, 1998). These approaches can be usefully employed by staff when offering bereavement support. Staff trained in the use of Social Stories or Comic Strip Conversations (Gray, 1998) which are descriptive and visual methods for teaching people with high-functioning autism and Asperger syndrome, may find these skills useful when supporting bereaved clients at the able end of the spectrum.

Understanding individual clients

Personalities
It is impossible to offer effective support for a bereaved person with autism without understanding their individual personality. This knowledge can be acquired only over a period of time by caring for them and observing them carefully, by having a continuing dialogue with parents and by consultation with staff who previously cared for them. Staff should also familiarise themselves with the client's life story and past experiences. It is worth remembering that people with autism differ from each other more than those not so affected as noted by Rita Jordan at The National Autistic Society Annual General Meeting in 1998, possibly because they are likely to be unresponsive to social influences.

Previous losses: impact on subsequent bereavements
Staff need to be sensitive to the fact that previous losses and bereavements may interact with a subsequent bereavement. The subsequent bereavement may reactivate the pain of earlier loss which may actually be felt for the first time, because it may never have been resolved (Worden, 1991). It is therefore important for staff to learn as much as possible about previous losses and bereavements of those in their care, when they happened, how they were managed by carers and how the individual reacted. Consultation with parents and staff who have cared for them in the past can be helpful.

The types of losses likely to have been experienced by adults with autism are listed in Part I and may include losses other than the death of someone close, such as those resulting from life transitions and staff changes.

Significant facts
It is also important to have easily accessible and specific personal information on each client's file, not only for general purposes, but also necessary at the time of a bereavement. This information should include:
- the cultural and religious beliefs and traditions of the client's family
- the contact details of interested family members and other important people in the client's life (such as family friends, a citizen advocate or 'befriender')
- the contact details of the client's social worker, doctor and other involved professionals.

Possession of these facts can be helpful when the staff need to take practical measures following the death of a client or of a client's family member, and/or notifying people who need to be informed of the death. The bereavement questionnaire can be a useful device in assembling these details.

Forms of address

It is essential for the effective management of bereavement that staff have access not only to the names, addresses and relationships of interested family members, but also a note of how they are addressed by the person with autism. It is no good consoling an individual for the death of 'Dad' if he was known as 'Father', 'Nan' if she was known as 'Granny', 'Mum' if she was known as 'Mummy' or of 'Catherine' if she was known as 'Kate.'

Religious and cultural backgrounds

An understanding of the religious and cultural tradition of the clients is essential for staff involved in the management of bereavement. This will help them confidently and sensitively to support a bereaved client in the grieving process by drawing on concepts acceptable to the family and from the client's own upbringing. Staff can prepare a client for what to expect in the rituals surrounding bereavement and, where necessary, accompany him or her to the funeral and other ceremonies. When a client dies, staff may need to be involved in making arrangements for the funeral or a memorial service.

Staff may therefore need to seek information on religious and cultural customs and rituals from family members of clients and also local ministers of religion, rabbis or leaders of other religious groups. They are likely to discover that such people are pleased to be of help.

Religion and cultural topics are included in *Understanding Grief* (Sheila Hollins and Lester Sireling, 1999) an in-house training course for those caring for people with learning disabilities who have been bereaved. A useful book covering rites, rituals and mourning traditions for the major religious and secular belief systems is *Death and bereavement across cultures* (Eds. Colin Murray Parkes, Pittu Laugani and Bill Young, 1997) (see References).

Information on humanist and non-religious funerals and cremations can be obtained from the British Humanist Association or the National Secular Society (see Useful Addresses).

Training staff to provide loss and death education for service users

Compared to the training resources on the management of bereavement, there are comparatively few aimed at providing education about loss and death so that people can be prepared to manage their own feelings in the event of future bereavements. Among them are the following:
- *Good Grief* (2) (Barbara Ward et al, 1996) a manual designed for 'exploring feelings, loss and death with over elevens and adults'
- *Undertaking Grief* (Sheila Hollins and Lester Sireling, 1999) a training course for working with people who have learning disabilities
- *Talking with Children and Young People about Death and Dying* (Mary Turner, 1998) a workbook designed for use with individual children and young people or with groups in a supportive setting only.

All of these, especially *Talking with Children and Young People about Death and Dying*, can be adapted to people with autism. In addition it is well worth reading 'Communicating about loss and mourning' in *Mental Retardation* (Yanok and Beifus, 1993), which describes a curriculum 'designed and field tested on a sample of verbally expressive adults with mental retardation.' Although it is unlikely that a curriculum modelled on the one described would be appropriate for most people with autism because of the breadth of the spectrum and their high anxiety levels, a number of the ideas on which it is based may be helpful.

Preparing people with autism for loss and bereavement

Need for preparation
Education about loss and death for children and people with learning disabilities, when developmentally appropriate, helps to make it less difficult for them to deal with bereavement when the time comes (Ward et al, 1996, Hollins and Sireling, 1999). The same applies to people with autism as part of their right to share in normal experiences. This preparation must be undertaken with caution and an understanding of the individual concerned.

Because of the individuality of people with autism, their varying levels of cognitive impairments, emotional immaturity and high levels of anxiety, it is likely that the preparation will need to take place informally, on an individual basis and when appropriate opportunities present themselves.

Saying goodbye: endings and new beginnings

Staff know the importance of preparing people with autism for the losses which can occur in everyday life so that having handled these 'little deaths', they may become more able to cope with major bereavements. They will need to be made aware of saying goodbye to things and people in their lives and of responding positively to new situations. Some clients find it difficult to part from their families at the end of home visits and they should be helped to overcome their distress by being encouraged to look forward to pleasurable activities on their return to their care unit, as well as to think about future home visits.

Another common loss in services for people with autism is the departure of staff. This can provide opportunities for the rituals of farewell such as parties and gifts. It can be argued that because of the effects on clients, staff should be careful not to let ties become too strong but if the ties are those of friendship with no pathological overtones, discouraging them will deprive clients of real life experiences.

Opportunities can be provided for maintaining contact with staff who have left by telephone calls, letters and visits and it can be pointed out to clients how these actions help to convert loss into gain.

Memory Books

Those clients who are capable of doing so and for whom it is appropriate might be encouraged to compile 'Memory Books' or 'Life Story Books' which are visual records of experiences which have been important to them. Parents and other significant people should be invited to contribute. They could include pictures of happy incidents in their lives, family holidays, previous homes, letters and postcards from home and photographs of family members and pets at different stages of their lives. As well as from giving pleasure during moments of relaxation, these books, with assistance from staff, may help clients to understand the concepts of the flow of life and of ageing. They may help with the grieving process in due course, and with learning that reminiscences about family members or pets who have died can be rewarding.

As part of this exercise, videos of family activities might be helpful, but should be used with caution. They may confuse the client about the finality of death if the people appearing in them have subsequently died.

Explaining death to people on the autistic spectrum

Opportunities should be taken to explain death simply and factually, as part of the life cycle, without speculation or prediction. Examples used can be occurring in daily life, such as dead plants, dead insects and dead animals to explain the concept of biological death. It is thought that children who have been prepared with a good biological explanation of death may be able to accept and understand the concept of an after-life (Schaeffer and Lyons, 1988). This may also be true of people with autism.

Opportunities can also be taken to comment on the deaths of people not close to them, such as public figures or acquaintances. There may be circumstances when it is appropriate for them to write letters of condolence or to send flowers to bereaved people who are in their circle of friends or acquaintances.

It is likely that many people with autism will have difficulty in grasping the components of the concept of death: inevitability – the realisation that life comes to an end; irreversibility – the permanence of death; non-functionality – the body ceasing to function and universality – the fact that it happens to all living creatures. (*Booklet 3*, Cathcart, 1994, Kane, 1997).

All of the world religions believe in the continuation of the soul after death: Hindus, Buddhists and Sikhs believe in reincarnation (that the soul returns as a new person many times). Christians, Jews and Moslems believe that a person lives only once and that after death their soul will go to heaven or hell.

Staff themselves may be uncertain whether the death of a person is the final end or whether there is such a thing as immortality. *Good Grief* (2) (Ward 1998) advises that it is better to say that 'no one yet knows', but that people are still trying to find out than to say to say 'I don't know.' Staff with strong religious beliefs or strong atheist convictions must recognise that these are their own personal views and not permit them to distort their professionalism in supporting the bereaved.

Good Grief (2) includes a very good section in which beliefs about death are simply explained. This can be summarised as follows and made appropriate for people on the autistic spectrum:

There are two aspects of death, the body and the spiritual aspect.

The body
What happens to the body can be understood by children if it is explained simply – that the dead person cannot have feelings, cannot feel hot or cold, hurt or sick. His dead body is of no use to him. A simple explanation is then given of cremation and burial.

The spiritual aspect
The following ideas are considered:
1. There is no continuance of the individual spirit

2. There is a continuation in some form. People die when they have done the work they have to do, but life may continue in a different way. Some children have found the concept of the lifecycle of insects helpful (see *Waterbugs and Dragonflies* by Doris Stickney, 1984) or even the concept of the persistence of atoms and electrons after the cremation of the body
3. There are differing points of view on the religious aspects of the soul and spirit. Abstract religious ideas are not necessarily helpful and Christian concepts are particularly difficult to understand. Children find it easier to come to terms with pantheism and reincarnation.

The chapter goes on to discuss three aspects of death of particular concern to children, which can be adapted for people with autism as appropriate:
1. Are dead people sleeping? A clear distinction should be made between sleep and death. Sleep gives rest and renewal. Death is when the body stops working.
2. What happens to dead people? Our bodies wear out. Our spirit or soul, which enables us to give and receive love never wears out. We cannot see it, but people of all religions believe it lives on after we die. The analogy is offered of a person leaving a house, which then ceases to be a home.
3. What is heaven like? The spirit or soul no longer experiences the sadness and troubles we have on earth. It goes to heaven which is where God is. Because God is love, heaven is a place full of love. No-one knows what heaven looks like or where it is (Hayworth, 1996).

It may be that these concepts are too difficult for many people with autism to understand. The most effective explanations of death are those which are simple and which draw as far as possible on the individual's own experiences. Their level of understanding must dictate the pace. It must be borne in mind, however, that introducing discussion which will cause anxiety in a person with autism is counter-productive. It is important, too, that when discussing concepts of death, staff must be careful not to confuse clients with ideas which might conflict with their cultural backgrounds.

Anxiety and misconceptions about death

People with autism may become fearful and anxious about death. This anxiety may arise in different ways. They may be unconcerned about the death of older people such as grandparents, but anxious when they hear of deaths in their own age groups. If they have lost one member of the immediate family, especially a parent, they may be fearful of losing remaining family members. They may feel threatened by deaths represented on television. Staff may find that they need to reassure those in their care, playing down the likelihood of imminent death of the client or of family members or, if appropriate, drawing on the concepts of the continuation of life in some form. There is a particular need for staff to be vigilant in regard to high-functioning people with autism, and especially those with Asperger syndrome, who may become obsessed with the idea of death and even of taking their own lives.

People with autism can have bizarre and distorted ideas of death. If staff detect misunderstanding about death, they should try to clarify its source and nature by sensitive questioning and observation, in order to tackle it effectively. An example of how this type of misunderstanding can arise is that of a young school leaver who was convinced that his own death was imminent. He knew that a member of staff had died and had therefore left the premises; he had also watched older pupils depart, never to be seen again. When staff discovered the source of his anxiety, they were able to arrange for him to speak to those pupils who had left, who told him about their life in a new setting.

Training staff to support clients when bereavement occurs

Effective support for bereaved clients relies in the first instance on staff understanding the common responses to bereavement and causes of grief. They can then relate these factors to the grieving processes of individual clients and how they are affected by autism with regard to their position on the spectrum.

There are now a wide variety of training resources available (see also References) within the following categories with examples given in brackets:
- standard books on bereavement (Parkes, 1996; Worden, 1991)
- a book offering guidance for those supporting survivors of suicide (Wertheimer, 1991)
- bereavement in children and young people (Ward et al, 1996)
- general training in bereavement support (the local branch of CRUSE, the bereavement care organisation, might be willing to provide a speaker or discussion group leader)
- bereavement in people with learning disabilities (three booklets by Cathcart, 1994, and Hollins and Sireling, 1999)
- bereavement in people with autism (chapter on 'Attachment and Loss' in Morgan, 1996)
- training in bereavement care of people with learning disabilities (the British Institute of Learning Disabilities can assist in this – see Useful Addresses)

- training in bereavement care of people with autism (consult The National Autistic Society – see Useful Addresses).

In-house training is recommended because it can enable staff to plan together as a team (*Booklet 3*, Cathcart, 1994). It is important for services to build up their library of helpful books and pamphlets. The local branch of CRUSE can provide a comprehensive list of publications.

When a death affects a service for adults with autism, staff will inevitably be under pressure to make decisions, to take action and to offer comfort. Furthermore, they may be suffering personal distress due to their own feelings of bereavement. Appropriate training, therefore, will enable staff to react with competence and sensitivity when they find themselves suddenly confronted with the problems which accompany such a death. It is important that there should always be staff available who have received bereavement training and to review this training periodically.

PART III

Supportive measures for bereaved people with autism

Designating members of staff to support bereaved clients

One of the functions of a bereavement support group is 'to ensure that clients are supported during their grieving by designated members of staff who understand the grieving process.' Decisions regarding those who should undertake this role in regard to individual clients should be preceded by consultations with those who know them best, including family members if possible. If a death is anticipated, advantage should be taken of the extra time to select suitable staff for this role and to remind them of the problems which may be involved.

The relationship to the client and the ability to feel comfortable when talking about death are the most important factors in the selection of a member of staff to support a bereaved client.

Ideally, the key worker, assisted by another staff member who knows the client well, would serve in this capacity, but there may be good reasons why certain individuals may not wish to undertake this role, such as a lack of experience of bereavement, or concern that a bereavement experience of their own might be brought to the surface again. No-one who has suffered a recent bereavement should be called upon to support a bereaved client. A bereavement support worker need not necessarily be a member of the care staff. They could be a member of the maintenance or office staff with whom the client has a particular affinity.

The bereavement support worker should be prepared:
- to keep all staff who come into contact with the client informed of their reactions to the bereavement and of their special needs deriving from it
- to enable the client to participate in the rituals surrounding death, preferably with the agreement of the client's family
- to comfort the bereaved and facilitate the grieving process.

It is recognised that because of staff rotas, it is not possible for the support worker, or even the person who assists them, to be on duty at all times during the bereavement process, which may last more than two years. Staff caring for the bereaved client must have access at all times to a member of staff, preferably a member of the bereavement support group, who can provide them with support and guidance.

Anticipated or sudden death: informing the client

Anticipated death

Although it is not conclusive, there is some evidence that if death is anticipated, the grieving process is less difficult for the bereaved than in the case of sudden death (Parkes, 1996). Anticipated death can lead to pre-death bereavement and can also be a source of acute anxiety (Worden, 1991). Staff will therefore wish to consider carefully, in the light of their knowledge of the client's personality, whether or not they should be informed of the impending death and, if at all possible, to discuss the matter with the family before making a decision. One young man with autism who knew that his father had a weak heart was able to accept the fact of his death when he was told that this father had died of a heart attack, although he suffered acute grief reactions.

Visiting the dying

Giving a client the opportunity to visit the dying relative in hospital and to say goodbye may help him or her to accept the finality of death and play a positive role in the grieving process (see Hollins and Sireling, 1999, *When Dad Died*, in which a son visits his dying father). Staff will wish to discuss with the family whether it is in the client's interest to visit, bearing in mind that some might find the occasion unduly stressful or a source of anxiety. It may be unwise to plan a visit if the patient is on drips or receiving visible life support. If it is agreed that the client should visit, care preparation should be made, such as ensuring that the staff member escorting the client is confident of carrying out the difficult task of visiting someone who is terminally ill. Briefing the client is also important so that he or she will know what to expect, possibly discussing any changes such as the dying person becoming weaker or unable to communicate (*Booklet 3*, Cathcart, 1994).

Staff should remember that the visit need not be a long one and that conversation is not necessary. The client can sit beside the patient, perhaps taking his or her hand. It may be appropriate to encourage the client to give the dying person a present as long as they are made to realise that this will not enable them to recover, but that the gift will be appreciated (*Booklet 3*, Cathcart, 1994).

Sudden death

Sudden death can devastate a service. Those affected suffer profound shock; they experience the natural stages of grief but in a more acute and amplified form.

Small services are particularly vulnerable and need access to an independent support network of those who are themselves not grieving. Staff and residents are likely to find it particularly difficult to re-enter the home, particularly the room of the deceased. Some staff may have anxieties about undertaking sleeping-in duties and some residents may need to take comfort in room-sharing for a period.

It is vitally important that news of the death is communicated speedily to all who are likely to be affected by it, for example, other service users, staff, parents and involved professionals. It is imperative that all are informed directly and do not learn from hearsay. The service should be prepared to offer support and reassurance to all those affected by the death. (For advice on how to break the news, see below)

A sudden death is likely to lead to a post-mortem and inquest. If this is the case, there will be a delay before funeral arrangements can be finalised. This will be a period of disquiet for everyone affected, especially those who were providing 'hands-on' care.

In the main, this section refers to the death of a client but there are common principles which would equally apply to the sudden death of a staff member or parent.

Initiating bereavement management

Who should tell the client of the death?

The decision about who should inform the client of the death should be thought through carefully. Should a client on the autistic spectrum be told by someone in the family, or by a staff member? If the death is that of a family member or someone close to the family, the decision should be reached in consultation with the family. There are examples of parents unwilling to tell their son or daughter of the death of someone close in order to avoid the devastating impact on them but, however well-intentioned, the withholding of information cannot be considered good practice.

It is possible that the bearer of the news may become the client's target of aggression in an expression of anger characteristic of bereavement, so it may be unwise, for example, to permit a mother living on her own to undertake this task. For the same reason, if a member of staff is selected to inform the client, it might not be appropriate for the same person to be the client's support-worker throughout the grieving process. When breaking the news, the informant should be supported by another staff member and a quiet location should be chosen where there will be no interruptions.

How to inform the client

Staudacher (1988) gives some practical advice on how to inform a child about death, which are adapted here for people with autism.
- Use forms of communication appropriate for the level of clients' understanding.
- Tell the truth, without giving unnecessary or disturbing details.
- Do not expect clients to respond in a way 'acceptable' to staff – with overt sadness.
- Observe how they appear to be feeling.
- Allow clients to release their feelings.
- Allow clients to take the lead and ask questions (in some circumstances they may need sensitive prompting).
- Answer all questions readily and honestly. If there is no answer, say 'No one knows' and if an answer is not immediately available, undertake to obtain it as soon as possible.
- Reassure clients that their life's routine in the establishment will go on and that they will continue to be cared for (bearing in mind that home visits may have to cease).
- Show affection and support.

Terms in which the death should be explained

A simple, factual description of death is recommended for both children and those with learning disabilities (Schaeffer and Lyons, 1988, Hollins and Sireling, 1999) along the lines of :

His/her body won't work any more. It can't move, talk, walk, see or hear. He/she is not asleep, has stopped breathing, can't eat, drink, feel hot or cold.

There should be no suggestion that there is hope of return (but see mention of reincarnation below) and euphemisms such as 'gone to sleep', 'left us,' and 'you have lost your father/mother' should be avoided as they may lead to confusion and distress. In some cases, it may be helpful to use the technique of asking the client to repeat what they have been told. Any misapprehensions about nature and cause of death should be cleared up immediately. For example, after his father's death, one school age boy developed an obsession for rushing upstairs wherever he was, in order to get to the attic or roof space. It transpired that his brother, when talking about his father's death, had pointed upwards and said that he was 'up there.' The boy had interpreted this to mean that his father was in the attic (Jordan and Powell, 1985).

This tendency of people with autistic spectrum disorders, especially those with Asperger syndrome, to interpret things literally must always be taken into account. The impression that the deceased 'has gone to a better place' should be avoided and it should be made clear that living is truly desirable. A doctrinaire stance is necessary in this instance to prevent preoccupation with suicide (Rawlings, 1998).

The ability of the client to understand accurately what they are told about death may affect their ability to work through the normal grieving process (McLoughlin, 1986). Staff can help by doing everything in their power to give clients an understanding of the death at a level at which it can be absorbed. Viewing the body can be the most effective means of accomplishing this. One young woman without speech, who was taken to view her mother's body after death, appeared to understand immediately the irreversibility of death. Having been unable to wake her mother, she sighed, 'empty, all gone.' Maureen Oswin describes how a profoundly disabled young woman without speech was helped to learn about her mother's death by being shown a photograph of her previously deceased father and by being given her mother's clothes to handle (Oswin, 1991). For non-verbal clients the use of signs, symbols and photographs can be useful in explaining a death. For example, a service which kept a correspondence file with photographs of family and friends helped one client to accept the death of his grandmother by transferring her photographs from the file to a special album.

The terms in which death is explained to the client should be discussed with the family and every effort should be made to comply with their wishes. This advice may run counter to the recommendation of a purely factual explanation of death, but if the family wish the client to be told the deceased 'has gone to heaven' or 'is with Jesus', this wish should be respected, although it should be pointed out that confusion may arise if the client should view the body or attend the funeral, cremation or burial. There are examples, however, of successful resolution of grief by people with autism who have been told that the deceased has gone to heaven, and subsequently participated in the bereavement rituals. Some clients have seemed to accept 'gone to heaven' as a factual explanation of someone having gone to a specific place where they themselves cannot at present go. Others have found comfort in the concept of reincarnation. There is no doubt that a number of people with autism have derived benefit from after-life beliefs (see Appendices).

If the client has experienced a previous bereavement, it is important to explain any subsequent death in the same terms. Again, the family may need to be consulted.

Explaining the cause of death

The four categories of death – natural, accidental, suicidal and homicidal – and the type of death can all have an effect on the grieving process (Worden, 1991). The first two types of death are more easily explained to the person with autism. People with autism sometimes ask where or when a person died, but seldom ask how, although staff should be prepared for them to do so. Those who do ask 'how' may be better able to assimilate the answer.

In explaining death, it is important always to be honest and consistent, without giving details which are unnecessary or disturbing (Staudacher, 1988). The cause of natural death can be explained by saying that the deceased 'was very old so that his/her) body wore out and stopped working (Schaeffer and Lyons, 1998) or that they were 'fatally' (or 'terminally') ill, 'and the doctor could not make them better.' Care should be taken, when mentioning illness, to avoid using the expression 'very ill' which might later be used on occasion when the client is ill, leading them to believe that they themselves are on the point of death.

An accidental death can be explained by saying that 'his/her body was so badly hurt that the doctor could not make it better, so it stopped working' (Schaeffer and Lyons, 1998).

Bereavement advice concerning the impact on children of death by suicide emphasises that they should be told the truth simply and honestly. Experience has shown that they are likely to find out indirectly or to realise that they are not being told the truth, with severe adverse consequences to themselves in either case. If there is no doubt that the deceased planned to kill themselves, the death should be explained to a child along the following lines: 'Sometimes a person's mind doesn't work right. They can't see things clearly and they felt the only way to solve their problems was by ending their life' (Schaeffer and Lyons, 1998). This might not be an appropriate explanation to offer to a person with autism. The more able person with autism is more likely than the majority to ask how the death occurred and might even ask if it was done on purpose. On the other hand, there are dangers in informing them of suicide because there is a high level of severe depression in this group, sometimes leading to suicide. It is strongly recommended that if the person with autism is told that their family member has committed suicide, specialised counselling help should be sought, and made available throughout the bereavement period.

If the bereaved client is in residential care, has a very limited capacity for understanding, and is highly unlikely to find out about, be informed of, or even comprehend the notion of suicide, it is recommended that the cause of death not be mentioned.

Should it be necessary to speak of the mode of death, the explanation should be confined to the minimum of necessary information such as 'they took too many pills, which made them fatally ill and the doctor couldn't make them better' (overdose), 'a train ran over them and their body was so hurt and broken that it can't work anymore' (threw themselves under a train), or 'their body was so hurt and broken, it can't work anymore' (hanging).

It cannot be overemphasised that if a client loses someone close to them by suicide, staff should assess the whole situation carefully. They must be particularly sensitive and discreet if the client is at the able end of the autistic spectrum.

Much of the above advice applies equally to homicide. Specialist counselling help should be sought if at all possible.

Deciding who will inform other parties of the bereavement

If possible, staff should discuss with the surviving members of the client's family who should take responsibility for informing those who need to be told of the bereavement, such as the client's advocate or befriender, their doctor and social worker, whose names, addresses and telephone numbers should already be easily accessible on the client's file.

All staff members who are likely to come in contact with the bereaved client should be informed quickly and privately. So that absolute consistency can be maintained in the management of the bereavement, staff should be told of any significant factors relating to it, such as:

- the relationship of the client to the deceased, both familial and emotional (whether close and whether contact was frequent and regular, for example)
- if the death was anticipated, whether the client was aware of this
- the terms in which the death was explained to the client, and how the client reacted
- whether the client will participate in the rituals surrounding bereavement
- previous losses suffered by the client.

Decisions will need to be made whether to tell other clients about the bereavement, and if so, in what terms.

Participation in rituals surrounding death

It is recognised that participation in the rituals surrounding death can help in the grieving process for those without learning disabilities. It provides an opportunity to face the reality of the death, to begin to come to terms with it, to say farewell to the deceased, and to share grief with others. It is now accepted, too, that most people with learning disabilities should be offered the opportunity to participate in the bereavement rituals and this is no less true for people with autistic spectrum disorders. Accordingly, unless the bereaved client has expressed a clear wish not to participate in these rituals, staff should be prepared to arrange for him or her to view the body of the deceased and to attend the funeral. Clients should not be excluded because it is thought they would not understand or might be upset.

Staff should give clear advice to the family along these lines and they should always ensure that one or two staff members who know the client well accompany the client on these occasions so that the family members, who may be seriously distressed by their own grief, need not be responsible for them.

On the other hand, there may be good reasons why the client should not participate in some of the rituals (such as viewing the body or attending the funeral) or there may be strong family objections to their doing so, and these views must be considered.

If a client is to be present at any of the rituals surrounding death, it is essential that staff make it quite clear what they should expect. If possible, it may be helpful for staff to gain as much information as they can, either from family members, the priest, or religious leaders. It is valuable, if time allows, to visit or take the client to visit relevant locations in advance of the funeral – the church, synagogue, temple, mosque, cemetery or crematorium. Clients who regularly attend a place of worship should be warned that expected rituals may not occur during the funeral service.

It may be of help to the client to describe the actions of the mourners at a funeral (singing hymns, saying prayers for the deceased, the fact that the priest or religious leader may speak about the deceased), the meanings of the rituals (as far as they can be understood by the client), and the fact that the body (inside the coffin) will be moved to the front in the ceremony. The client should also be told that it is all right to cry at a funeral.

Viewing the body

Viewing the body can help the bereaved understand the finality of death. If it is agreed that the client should view the body, it is important that they should be told what to expect, for example, that it will be cold to touch. Care should be taken to ensure that they are made aware that the whole body is there. Children, seeing only the head of the deceased in the coffin, have been known to conclude that it has been severed from the body (Schaeffer and Lyons, 1998). It is possible that a person with autism may think this, too. In some instances, therefore, it could be helpful for the client to touch the body.

However, viewing the body should be avoided if it is likely to cause distress to the client. The client's expressed reluctance or the nature of his or her temperament may make this inadvisable. Similarly, if the body has been mutilated in some way it may not be an appropriate course of action.

Funeral

If possible, staff should agree with the family beforehand where they and the client should sit in the church, synagogue, temple or mosque. It may be wise for them to sit at the back so that they can make an inconspicuous exit if the client becomes distressed. The coffin and the fact that it is holding the body should be pointed out to the client. If flowers are an acceptable part of the culture, it would be wise to have encouraged the client to bring flowers to place on the coffin and they should be allowed to touch it.

Burial

If the body is to be buried, it should be made clear to the client that it will be protected from mud and rain by the coffin. The client may wish to join the other mourners in throwing a handful of earth on the coffin.

Cremation

If the body is to be cremated, the process of cremation should be explained to the client and they should be reassured that the deceased will suffer no pain as they are no longer able to feel anything.

Visiting the grave or memorial stone

Even if the client has not participated in other rituals, staff should try to arrange a visit to the grave or memorial stone, as this can be a helpful way for the client to say farewell to the deceased. The significance of the grave or the memorial stone should be explained to the client in terms they can understand. They could be encouraged to make some gesture, such as buying and placing flowers by the stone or planting a tree or rose bush. It may be appropriate to arrange further visits, particularly if the client requests it. Visits to the grave or memorial stone may help clients to come to terms with their bereavement. Consideration should be given to whether they could visit it on the anniversary of the death, or on other anniversaries, as a way of remembering the deceased. It is desirable to keep the surviving family members informed of these visits, but their permission is not essential.

Memorial service

Some families, particularly if the deceased has been of some prominence in the community, organise a memorial service, usually some weeks after the burial. It may not be appropriate for the bereaved client to attend the service because of the large number of people present. However, if the family expresses a wish for the client to attend, or if the client wishes to do so, staff should be prepared to explain the significance of the service and to accompany the client.

Mementoes

One strategy for helping clients to come to terms with a bereavement, if home visits are to cease, is arranging for them to visit the family home in order to choose objects which are significant for them. Clients can take these back to their living unit as mementoes which can give them a sense of continuity.

Comforting the bereaved (see Appendices for individual reactions to bereavement)

The impairments of communication and social interaction of people with autistic spectrum disorders may make it difficult for staff to discover whether or not grieving is taking place after bereavement, bearing in mind that it may be absent or delayed. If staff consider that it is taking place, they must be careful to ensure that the timing and duration of the grieving process and the 'tasks of mourning' are determined by the bereaved. In comforting the bereaved they must use the forms of communication, verbal, non-verbal or both in combination, which are best understood by them. The role of staff, which must be adapted to the personality of the bereaved, is to facilitate the grieving process by such measures as:

- being there when needed
- sensitive observation and knowing when to intervene
- explaining the grieving process at an appropriate level
- listening to and observing non-verbal expressions of grief (for physical and behavioural see subsequent paragraphs on grief reactions)
- asking how the client feels and supplying words to help, being careful not to plant ideas
- talking about the deceased and experiences they shared with the bereaved
- offering emotional support
- offering comfort in ways which the bereaved will accept, for example, physical contact such as touching, holding or massage
- ensuring that the bereaved is comfortable and not in physical pain or distress
- if it is compatible with a client's religious and ethnic background, and acceptable to the family, introducing references to after-life belief

- offering reassurance that life's routines will go on and that s/he will continue to be cared for
- ensuring that the bereaved has a quiet place in which to grieve if s/he indicates the need.

Facilitating access to therapeutic measures

In addition, the support workers' role is to provide the bereaved with access to any therapeutic measures which might meet their particular needs. They should not hesitate to seek specialist psychiatric, psychological or therapeutic support for the bereaved if they consider it necessary, but should bear in mind that such support can not only be ineffective but actually harmful if the practitioner does not have specific knowledge about autistic spectrum disorders. There is evidence that the psychodynamic/psychoanalytic approach can have seriously adverse effects on them (Gerland, 1999; Wolff, 1995).

Listed below are a selection of therapeutic measures, some of which will also be mentioned in the context of specific reactions to bereavement.
- counselling* (McCormick, 1998; Tantam, 2000)
- cognitive behaviour therapy* (Attwood, 1998; Prior, 2000)
- social stories* (Attwood, 2000; Gray, 1998)
- participation in an appropriate support group* (McCormick, 1998)
- medication (Tantam, 2000)
- opportunities for vigorous exercise (Attwood, 1993)
- relaxation techniques
- non-compulsive activities.

These measures can be helpful in alleviating anxiety and depression, conditions which are frequently associated with autism and may be exacerbated by bereavement. Those indicated with an asterisk may be appropriate only for people with high-functioning autism or Asperger syndrome.

Counselling intervention needs to be carefully planned in advance. This will involve assessment of the individuals and their degree of language competence as well as identifying the type of language, focus and structure appropriate to the particular circumstances (Tantam, 2000; McCormick, 1998).

Cognitive behaviour therapy, which can enable the client to learn strategies for dealing with particular social and emotional problems, requires the expertise of a clinical psychologist who is able to adapt it for use for people with autism spectrum disorders (Attwood, 1998; Prior, 2000). Described as 'applied common sense', it can be a helpful intervention in the context of a bereavement.

Social Stories are a strategy developed for people with high-functioning autism and Asperger syndrome in order to improve their understanding of social situations and offer them specific behaviours to use when interacting with others (Attwood, 2000; Gray, 1998). In the context of bereavement, they can be helpful in providing coping strategies and an understanding of other people's reactions to the bereavement (Attwood, personal communication, 1999). Written according to specific guidelines, they were initially used mainly for children, but they have been successfully adapted for use with adults. Staff wishing to learn how to use this strategy should read the chapter by Carol Gray, who developed it, in *Asperger syndrome or high-functioning autism?* (Gray, 1998).

It is essential, if medication is to be used, that the prescribing doctor is aware of the idiosyncratic reactions of people with autism and Asperger syndrome (Tantam, 2000). Staff may find that they need to be proactive in offering advice on the basis of their knowledge of the previous reactions of individuals in their care to drug therapy.

Facilitating supportive relationships

If neither parent is now alive, staff should be actively involved in facilitating the supportive relationships – such as successor parents and citizen advocates – which may have been arranged by the parent for their family member. The performance by the successor parent of at least some of the functions (for example, telephone calls, home visits and outings) for which the parents were previously responsible, can be very reassuring to the bereaved client and staff will wish to support them in doing so. In the absence of such designated persons, staff may wish to identify people who will reliably perform these functions through organisations such as churches, advocacy or befriending groups, being careful to ensure that the appropriate checks are made and that the introduction of the client to the relationship is carefully managed.

Coping with grief reactions

Staff will wish to take particular note of the common reactions to bereavement listed in Part I so they will have some idea of what the bereaved client may be feeling. It is helpful to focus on some of these reactions so that it can be decided which kinds of supportive measures are best for the client.

It is important to bear in mind that a number of these reactions can derive from causes other than bereavement. A familiarity with the client and good powers of observation may help staff members to determine the causes of distress, but it is safe to assume that bereavement may be a powerful factor for two years or more after the death of someone close to them.

Anger

Anger may be directed at the person who has died if the client feels they have been abandoned by them. It may also be directed at the person who broke the news of the death, or it may be a generalised anger. Anger may also arise when activities provided by the deceased are no longer available. Staff should enable the client to express this anger without harming themselves or others, or damaging property. One young man with autism expressed his anger by breaking up the furniture in his room. Had those caring for him been better prepared, they might perhaps have been able to divert his anger into vigorous exercise - hitting cushions or a punch bag, knocking a ball about, or tearing up old telephone books.

Guilt

This may arise from the 'magical thinking' characteristic of young children who have been bereaved, and who think they might have caused the death by their own actions. Guilt is anger turned on oneself, but in people with autism it is often expressed as overt anger. Staff will wish to avoid suggesting to a client that they might have feelings of guilt, but if they have evidence that this is so, they should reassure the client that the death was inevitable and not caused by their own or any other individual's actions, being careful to use the same terms in which the death was originally explained.

One young man with Asperger syndrome said that he felt guilty after a death in the family because other family members made it clear that they considered his reactions to be inappropriate. He needed to be reassured that he should not feel guilty as he had not been aware of how people normally react to bereavement. This was further complicated because he had not been diagnosed at the time and his family were unaware of his need for help and understanding.

Anxiety, fear and panic

Anxiety, fear and panic are all common responses to bereavement. These feelings are likely to be heightened in people with autism, not only because of the loss of someone important in their lives who may have represented stability and security, but also because the changes which almost inevitably follow bereavement are likely to be very threatening to a person with autism. The bereavement may also give rise to a fear of their own death, possibly resulting in a fear of going to sleep, or a fear that other members of their family may also die.

It may be helpful to treat anxiety, which can be closely related to depression, with alternatives to medication, such as vigorous exercise and relaxation techniques. Severe anxiety can be treated by a clinical psychologist trained in cognitive behaviour therapy (Attwood, 1998), who should also have sufficient knowledge of autistic spectrum disorders to adapt it accordingly.

If it is considered necessary to resort to medication, it is essential that the prescribing doctor is thoroughly knowledgeable about which drugs are most appropriate for use by people with autism and Asperger syndrome (Tantam, 2000).

Staff must be prepared to provide constant reassurance and to alleviate some of the effects of bereavement by encouraging the successor parent, a befriender or other surviving members of the family to keep in close touch with the client. They could, perhaps, fulfil some of the caring functions previously undertaken by the deceased, such as taking the client out for meals or for home visits. It is important to convince the client that they will continue to be cared for and to provide the security afforded by maintaining the usual routines of daily life. Unless the client has expressed a positive wish for change, changes in the client's life should not be introduced during the period of bereavement.

Depression and despair

The bereaved client will feel the emptiness and pain of loss acutely, but on no account should staff try to 'jolly' them out of their grief. 'They kept wanting me to dance, but I was too sad to' was a poignant comment made by a bereaved person with learning disabilities (Oswin, 1991). Talking about the deceased, though it may temporarily exacerbate the grief, is considered necessary for recovery from bereavement (Carr, 1988). In order to assist this process, it is important for staff to learn something about the deceased – how they looked, their personality, the nature of their relationship with the client, and the activities they shared. It is also important to know the terms of endearment the deceased used for the bereaved. This information can not only help staff to encourage the bereaved to communicate their memories of the deceased, but it can enable staff to speak to the client of the deceased in terms which are meaningful to them and from which they may derive comfort. Because people with autism have difficulty in understanding and expressing their feelings, staff need to help them to do so, at a level which is appropriate to them.

It can be difficult to identify depression in a person with autism, even those with Asperger syndrome, who are known to be at high risk of suicide. Health care professionals may unfortunately be unaware of this high risk (McCormick, 1998). It is therefore up to service staff to be vigilant in detecting thoughts of suicide and to advocate active therapeutic measures to deter them. Specialised counselling by people familiar with autistic spectrum disorders can be helpful for people with Asperger syndrome, as can participation in an appropriate support group (McCormick, 1998). Psychiatric/psychological intervention may need to be sought for those suffering from prolonged depression. Again, as stated above, medication should be prescribed only by someone who has a thorough knowledge of the idiosyncratic reactions of people with autism and Asperger syndrome (Tantam, 2000).

Physical symptoms, such as pain, appetite disturbance, breathlessness and illness

The physical symptoms of bereavement can cause acute discomfort. It is now generally accepted that bereavement can be responsible for the beginning or relapse of genuine illness (Hollins and Sireling, 1999). One young woman with autism who lost her father suffered a serious and prolonged period of asthma combined with anorexia, when she had to be fed by hand. Of course, staff need to determine whether the illness has been triggered by a factor other than bereavement, such as the side effects of medication. Good food – especially soft food (yoghurt, soup, puréed foods) – and warm drinks can be a source of comfort. Assistance with eating may also be comforting.

It is important to remember that body temperature may drop because of bereavement and it is therefore necessary to ensure that the client is kept warm and comfortable.

Increased need for sleep, sleeplessness and hyperactivity

The bereaved may require more than the usual amount of sleep or, conversely, they may suffer from insomnia or hyperactivity. Staff will need to create a balance between these reactions and the maintenance of a stable routine.

Nightmares

Staff on night duty should be made aware not only of the risk of sleeplessness but also of the fact that the bereaved may have frightening and disturbing nightmares. One young woman with autism dreamed she was eating meat, which turned out to be her deceased brother. If the nightmares persist, extra staff may need to be on duty, as the bereaved should be wakened, helped out of bed, and given a warm drink. They may need someone to sit with them after they return to bed and while they go to sleep.

Regression and loss of skills

Emotional and physical regression, increased dependency and loss of skills are common reactions to bereavement by the learning disabled. They may become uncharacteristically incontinent or bedridden (Hollins and Sireling, 1999; *Booklet 3*, Cathcart, 1994). Those caring for bereaved people with autism should be aware of these possible reactions and it is strongly advised that any forms of assessment should be avoided during a period of bereavement, as it would result in an entirely abnormal reading.

Absence of grief following bereavement

It is now known that some people with autistic spectrum disorders do not mourn after losing someone close to them. This absence of the grieving process does not appear to be related to the cognitive level of the bereaved, nor does it necessarily result in long-term adverse effects. The few examples known to us do not justify an assumption that they do not have a capacity to feel emotion in another context.

If an individual does not exhibit grief in an expected way, it does not necessarily follow that they are not grieving. Before it can be concluded that a bereaved individual is not grieving, staff need to verify their conclusion by careful observation, sensitive questioning and checking on the behaviour of the individual in different settings (Brelstaff, 1984). Furthermore, it cannot be concluded from the fact that there has not been a reaction to one bereavement that there will be no reactions to subsequent bereavements, particularly that of a second parent, which may result in the cessation of home visits and the type of caring provided by a parent.

Problems encountered in bereavement of people with autism

It is essential that those offering support to a bereaved client have a good understanding of autism, but they must also know the client well and be skilled in observing and interpreting both their verbal and non-verbal reactions. The grieving process of people with autism is impeded by their difficulties with communication, social interaction and cognition. Staff need to be aware of some of the problems which may arise.

Delayed reaction to loss

Grief is often a delayed process for people with learning disabilities. They fail initially to understand the implications of their loss, but may come to feel the impact later (Kitching, 1987). One young woman with autism whose father died before Christmas accepted that she could not go home for the holiday, having been given a reason – that daddy had gone to heaven – but did not begin the grieving process until she went home the following Christmas and realised her father's absence. She then underwent a profound grieving process for a period in excess of two years.

Apparent failure to understand the irreversibility of death

The failure to understand the irreversibility of death is characteristic of young children with learning disabilities (Schaeffer and Lyons, 1998). This is also true of people with autism, although the apparent failure to understand may reflect a language difficulty rather than a difficulty of comprehension.

It is normal in the early stages of bereavement to behave as though the deceased is still alive or even present, and to experience difficulty in accepting the finality of death. It may be that the client's repeated questions about the return of the deceased after the funeral and burial or cremation are their way of coming to terms with the loss. They may feel a need to check the consistency of the replies they are given or their questions may be their way of showing that they need comfort and reassurance. One young man with autism, who attended his father's funeral and cremation, persisted for some time in asking when his father would return.

Uncertain and inappropriate responses to bereavement

There have been a number of examples of people with autism who have expressed uncertainty regarding how they should react to the death of someone close to them: 'Should I feel sad?', 'How sad should I feel?', 'Shall I cry?' Others have reacted by giggling at the funeral or at the grave – perhaps a reflection of this uncertainty. Some have appeared callous and unfeeling, which is very difficult for carers. One girl, following the death of her mother, immediately asked when her father planned to marry again. Some apparently callous comments can be the result of difficulties with verbal expression.

Because people with high-functioning autism and Asperger syndrome look normal and appear to converse normally, they are expected to act like other people and to reflect conventional emotions. In fact, they may lack the coping mechanisms for dealing with emotions in themselves or others, and they can therefore appear to be callous and unfeeling when a bereavement occurs. They are confused, anxious and unable to comprehend the perceptions that others have of them under these circumstances, being made to feel that they have done something wrong, yet having no idea of how to put it right. Social stories, an intervention for improving social skills through heightened social understanding, offer a strategy which can be helpful for bereaved clients by providing a script of what will happen and what they should say and do in the specific circumstances. This can alleviate their anxiety by giving them the security in knowing what their role should be and by providing information on what other people within the specific situation are thinking and feeling (Attwood, personal communication, 1999).

Disruptive or challenging behaviour

Because of impaired communication and interaction skills, the only way a bereaved person with autism may be able to express their grief is by disruptive or challenging behaviour. It is difficult for staff to discover whether this arises from fear, anger, anxiety, guilt or physical discomfort, all of which can accompany bereavement, or whether it arises from factors altogether unrelated to bereavement, for example, from effects of medication or distress caused by the behaviour of another client. By careful observation and sensitive questioning, if the client will tolerate it, staff may be able to discover the cause of the behaviour and what the client may be trying to communicate so that they make take whatever action is appropriate. It may help to encourage them to participate in some non-compulsive activity which they are known to enjoy or to become involved in relaxation (aromatherapy, massage, being in the sensory room) or alternatively to undertake some vigorous exercise such as using gym equipment, jogging or aerobics.

Medication for behavioural problems, particularly aggression, is never an effective long-term solution (Tantam, 2000). It is important to remember that even long after the loss has occurred, the client's behaviour can be affected by bereavement.

Self-injurious behaviour

Self-injury, which can take the form of head-banging, hand-biting or scratching themselves, arises, like challenging behaviour, from impaired communication and interaction skills. Like challenging behaviour it can signal distress following bereavement, caused by fear, anger or physical discomfort, or it can be used as a means of communication. It is well worth reading the analysis of the cause of self-injury and the strategies which can help to overcome it in *Why does Chris do that?* by Tony Attwood (see References).

The same measures referred to in the point about challenging behaviour above can be helpful in discovering the cause and taking the appropriate supportive action, as well as encouraging clients to participate in an enjoyable activity, some form of relaxation therapy or to undertake some vigorous exercise.

Limited means of expressing grief

It is generally agreed that people without learning disabilities who are bereaved find it helpful to talk to sympathetic family members and friends about the deceased and about their feelings. Grief counselling, proven to have a very positive effect on the grieving process, involves listening to the bereaved and responding reassuringly and supportively. These therapeutic strategies are not available to people with autism at the more disabled end of the spectrum, unless staff can enable them to express their thoughts and feelings by means of sensitive questioning and by supplying appropriate words, signs or pictures. Because of the demands it makes upon them, this kind of attention may be unwelcome to the bereaved, who may find it threatening. On the other hand, if grief is present and not expressed, it may go on at an unconscious level which can precipitate symptoms of unresolved grief, such as deep depression or neurosis.

Those at the able end of the spectrum, despite their ability to converse, may need help and support in expressing their reactions to bereavement, which may be complicated by their feelings of inadequacy in responding in ways expected by others. Carefully structured counselling can be an appropriate intervention for them, as may the use of social stories (see pages 24, 44 and 50).

Inability to request help

Because of their disabilities of communication and social interaction, people with autism are unlikely to seek support when they are anxious, depressed or unhappy. Again, it is necessary for staff to intervene sensitively. Although a minority of people with autism do not apparently grieve when they lose someone close, the majority experience the grieving process and require help in order to succeed in achieving a resolution of grief.

Limited number of relationships

Most people with autism, as a consequence of their disabilities, have comparatively few close relationships. Consequently, there may be a very substantial emotional investment in these relationships, with the result that when they are terminated by departure or death, the effect on the person with autism may be catastrophic. Because they have a limited network of concerned family and friends, they may find it difficult to perform one of the tasks of mourning which must be worked through if the grieving process is to be completed, i.e. to find a different place for the deceased in their emotional lives and reinvest in new relationships (Worden, 1991).

In common with others with disabilities, many people with autism are highly dependent for help on professional staff who may not be able to provide long-term emotional care or support. It is therefore essential that parents arrange for supportive relationships between their family member and whoever will take over the advocacy and caring roles after they are no longer able to perform them. (see Part II, page 20).

Preoccupation with deaths of people with no close ties
There are a number of examples of high-functioning people with autism or those with Asperger syndrome who are obsessively interested in deaths reported in the media and with whom they have no personal connection. One young man became preoccupied with the death of Diana, Princess of Wales, and a young woman, obsessively interested in firemen, exhibited signs of acute grief on hearing of the death of one killed while trying to rescue someone in the course of his duties.

Inability to seek activities which may help the grieving process
People without learning disabilities have access to a number of strategies which can help to mitigate their loss. They may turn to vigorous exercise, pursue their hobbies, seek social contacts, travel or listen to music. People with autism may not have the self-awareness, motivation or experience to seek activities which might be helpful to them, and often they do not have access to them without help from carers.

Introduction of undesirable habits or obsessions
Staff may need to intervene if undesirable habits or obsessions are introduced by the bereaved during their grieving process as a source of comfort as these may persist long after the period of grieving, to the detriment of the client.

Inability to predict future change
People with autism are unlikely to have an expectation that the pain and suffering which they are experiencing will eventually come to an end. They therefore lack yet another possible source of comfort. Staff should make every effort to explain

the grieving process to them, bearing in mind that the intensity and duration of their reactions should be determined only by the bereaved. One support worker, when asked by the bereaved, 'Have I finished being sad?' gave her permission to do so, thereby assisting her in the resolution of grief (Rawlings, 1996).

Difficulties with accepting the need to move on

In the instance of sudden death, because of the intensity of emotions and general trauma of those affected, staff should be especially vigilant in approaching specific areas of sensitivity, for example, the sorting and dispersal of personal possessions and rearranging the bedroom of the deceased. Staff need to be sensitive to the possibility that those affected by the sudden death of a carer or family member may experience difficulty in coming to terms with it and in moving on with their own lives.

Anniversaries

Staff should be reminded that bereaved clients may need special attention on the occasion of the anniversary of the death and also at times of festivities such as Christmas, Easter and birthdays, which they may have shared with the deceased.

Grief and growth

The ultimate aim of staff should not only be to enable clients to achieve a successful resolution of grief, but also to enable them to transform their experience into a source of strength for themselves and of benefit to others. There have been some very moving examples of this achievement among people with autism who, having experienced bereavement themselves, have offered comfort to other clients, staff and family who were undergoing a grieving process. This is a reminder of the opening quotation:

'There is no growth without pain and conflict and no loss that cannot lead to gain' (Pincus, 1961)

PART IV

Other aspects of bereavement support

Support for surviving family members

After the death of someone close to a client, particularly a family member, staff may find that they are in close touch with the surviving family members who are also mourning the deceased. Staff should be prepared to offer support to family members in the following ways:
- keeping them informed of the reactions of the bereaved client
- helping them to understand and come to terms with the reactions of the client, in particular:
  - inappropriate behaviour
  - apparently callous reactions
  - anger, especially if it is directed towards the surviving family members.

A surviving mother may be the focus of aggression from a bereaved client as she may be held responsible for the death by the client, especially if she informed the client of the death. However, no surviving family member should be deterred from visiting the client because of the possibility of being the target of aggression. Staff should be prepared to be present and to intervene to protect the visitor.

Support of staff caring for a bereaved client

One of the functions of a bereavement support group should be the support of staff caring for bereaved clients as this role can be a very demanding one, requiring concentrated attention and commitment. One cause of stress can be the difficulty of determining whether the reactions of the client are the result of their bereavement or of totally unrelated factors. The anger characteristic of the grieving process may be directed toward the staff member supporting them. The staff member may also be distressed by witnessing the grief reactions of the bereaved client. The support group should therefore ensure that the staff member has access to one of their members at all times, not only for specific advice, but also to provide an informed and sympathetic response when they need to talk about their own feelings.

Bereaved staff

Individual members of staff who are themselves suffering the effects of bereavement may wish to seek support from a member or members of the bereavement support group. Staff may wish to meet in a 'sharing group' where they can express their feelings about the deceased and their own bereavement reactions without fear of interruption or criticism and receive sympathetic support. The session might be introduced and led by a senior member of staff, a member of the clergy or a member of CRUSE, who would explain the purpose of the session and how it would be conducted. The session should be held in quiet, comfortable surroundings with pre-arranged times for beginning and ending, and should last not more than one hour.

Loss of client or staff member

The death of a client or staff member can be particularly devastating for a service for people with autism, because it may have a direct effect on a number of staff and clients. In order to cope with losses of this kind, staff need to be prepared to undertake many of the practical arrangements following a death, such as registration and funeral (see Part II, page 22).

Who to inform

All staff and those clients who are likely to be affected by the death in any way should be informed of the death of a client or staff member. It should be borne in mind that unusual circumstances can be detected by even some of the less able clients. This can lead to the development of misapprehensions, possibly causing them more distress than the truth. Whether clients should be informed as a group or individually depends on the relationship of the clients to the deceased and to each other. Families of clients likely to be affected should also be informed.

Supporting clients who are likely to grieve

It is important to identify those clients who are likely to grieve for the deceased and to appoint a bereavement support worker who can help them through the grieving process and enable them to participate in the rituals surrounding the death, as previously described.

Support for surviving family members of a deceased client

Staff may find that they are called upon to offer support to the surviving family members of deceased clients, especially if they are parents. The disability of autism, by its very nature, isolates the individual from other people, both because of the behaviour it causes and because its complexity makes it difficult for others to understand. Family members will therefore turn to staff, being perhaps the only people who knew and liked the client as an individual and who were sympathetic to their needs. One of the factors in the grieving process is the need to talk about the deceased. Staff are uniquely qualified to listen sympathetically to surviving family members and thereby help them to come to terms with their loss.

Support for survivors of suicide

If a client has taken their own life, both staff and surviving family members may find this particularly difficult to come to terms with and may need expert counselling. The book by Alison Wertheimer, *A special scar*, is helpful in explaining the experience of people bereaved by suicide (see References).

Memorial service or ceremony

The opportunity to say 'goodbye' during some form of ritual can be a great help in the grieving process. A memorial service for the deceased staff member or client, which those who knew them can help to organise and in which they can participate, together with family members of the deceased, can provide this opportunity. It also provides a means of recalling the life of the deceased in a positive way. The local vicar or other appropriate clergy can be asked to officiate and to advise on the form the service might take. Alternatively, or in addition, it may be desirable to have a formal ceremony such as setting up a bench, planting a tree or erecting a memorial stone. Advice on memorial stones can be obtained from the local branch of CRUSE, who can provide a list of addresses.

If a group is to attend a funeral or memorial service, they should not go out in a minibus as if on an outing. Despite the expense, care should be taken to arrive in a more respectful and appropriate manner (Oswin, 1991).

PART V

Support for the dying

Care of the dying

Palliative care is the term given to skills, procedures and practices developed mainly within the hospice movement. Its focus on relief of pain and reduction of fear, underpinned by sensitive communication with the patient, is particularly relevant to the care of the dying (Dickenson and Johnson, 1993). It is based on the care of the whole person, meeting the physical, psychological, social and spiritual needs of the dying and according them dignity and value (Peberdy, 1993).

For those cared for in services for adults with autism, there are three groups of people who would be involved in such palliative care of the dying:
- the care staff employed by the service;
- healthcare professionals, in particular nursing staff;
- the family of the patient.

If the relationship of these groups to each other is based on co-operation, mutual respect and good communication, this will have a positive impact on the quality of palliative care which they can deliver to the patient (Read, 1998).

Training for support staff

It is recommended that as part of bereavement training for staff in services for adults with autism, at least some staff should be trained in support for the dying, including the principles of palliative care. The Hospice Information Service is a helpful source of information on training, and the library at St. Christopher's Hospice in London has copies of articles on palliative care of people with learning disabilities which include information relevant to the needs of people with autism (see Useful Addresses). As with bereavement support, the approach to care of the dying needs to be unique to each individual, but certain principles apply to all.

Needs of support staff

It is important that the service caring for the person with autism who has a terminal illness should ensure the needs of staff supporting the patient are adequately met. For example, they may require:
- counselling or psychological support to enable them to manage their own feelings of fear and anxiety
- support regarding the process of breaking bad news
- advice on the process of communicating with the patient in order to minimise the risk of causing anxiety
- assistance in obtaining information on the medical needs of the patient and the course of the illness.

(Read, 1998)

Knowing the individual patient well

It is preferable that a small number of key support workers is dedicated to the care of the dying client, consistent with the availability of 24 hour support and, if at all possible, they serve in this capacity until the end. They should know the patient well, so the client will have complete confidence in them, and so that they will be able to interpret the patient's verbal and non-verbal reactions in order to ensure the patient receives the care he or she needs. Many people with autism will not openly indicate when they are feeling pain or discomfort. Support workers must therefore also be very observant, so that they can take appropriate measures to alleviate the client's anxiety and discomfort and advocate on their behalf to health care professionals.

Communication: the need for tranquillity and a consistent approach

It is absolutely vital to avoid anxiety reactions on the part of the client so that their mental tranquillity is maintained at all times. There must be consistency at all levels of care and communication so this can be achieved.

Support staff
Staff supporting the patient should have effective daily communication with each other, both regarding the care provided to the patient and what is said to them.

Uncertainty or inconsistency on the part of staff can be easily perceived by a person with autism and can lead to anxiety.

Health care professionals

Support staff will need to act as mediators between health care professionals and the patients to ensure effective communication between them and to ensure consistency in the information provided, as well as the wording employed.

Family and friends

Every effort should be made to ensure that family members and friends who visit the patient are in agreement with each other and with the staff on the type of support to be provided and on what information should be given to the patient about the illness.

Communication with the patient: the need for tact and care

The issue of how much information should be given to the dying can be determined only by a careful assessment of the individual and consultation both with support staff and those family members who wish to be involved. It is important that all those involved concentrate on providing a reassuring quality of life to the dying one day at a time, constantly bearing in mind the need to avoid any anxiety response.

Staff should learn about the symptoms and expected course of the illness of the patient they are supporting, communicating this information only if there are very positive reasons for doing so. Failure to provide answers to persistent questions from the patient will cause increased anxiety.

For many of those at the more disabled end of the spectrum, it is unlikely that providing them with information about the progression and outcome of their illness would be in their best interests. Although they may have some understanding of death, they may not be able to refer the process to themselves. Probing to find out about their perception of death may serve only to arouse their anxieties.

However, communicating information to more able individuals would need to be judged on the basis of an assessment of their understanding of their illness and its implications for their own death. The patient may need help and support in exploring their own feelings about dying, death and after-life beliefs. Carers must take the lead from the patient, while at the same time avoiding false hopes.

People with autism have difficulty accepting changes in routine, as well as uncertainty regarding both the short and long-term future. Staff who know the patient well will need to employ the coping strategies which have been successful in the past in order to maintain the patient's peace of mind. Some individuals with autism can at times simultaneously hold two incompatible ideas in their minds, a condition which has been observed occurring in people facing the prospect of death (Lansdown, 1996). Denial may also be a means of coping with the prospect of death.

It is strongly recommended that staff, especially those supporting able clients, read Part 3 of the book *Death, dying and bereavement* (edited by Dickenson and Johnson, 1993) entitled 'Caring for Dying People', so that they may be aware of strategies for dealing with uncertainty, denial and difficult questions raised by the dying.

The religious dimension

If the patient is associated with a religious community, staff should seek advice from the significant persons in that community about the importance placed on the rituals of dying and death. Most clergy are accustomed to supporting the dying and they could make a useful contribution to support for the patient provided that they are carefully briefed about the autistic dimension. Again it is strongly recommended that staff read the relevant chapters in *Death, dying and bereavement* (edited by Dickenson and Johnson, 1993). *Death and bereavement across cultures* (edited by Parkes et al., 1997) is also a useful book.

The patient's physical comfort

Attention to the patient's physical comfort includes not only pain control but also ensuring that the bed and sheets are comfortable and clean, that blankets are used so that the weight covering can be varied as necessary, and that the room temperature and ventilation are well maintained for the patient's optimum comfort. Consideration should be given to the use of complementary therapies which help to induce relaxation, such as massage and aromatherapy.

Appropriate diet

It is very important that the patient is provided with a diet appropriate to their appetite and health care needs, having regard not only to taste but also to consistency. Staff may need to help the patient to eat by encouraging them or by actually feeding them. This is particularly necessary in a hospital environment, where too many patients have been left undernourished because staff do not consider feeding them to be their responsibility.

Location

If possible, the dying person should be cared for in familiar, quiet and tranquil surroundings. Ideally, this should be either on the premises of the service which has provided residential care for them or, if they have been living independently, in their own home.

If care in a hospice is considered appropriate, or if the appropriate level of care can be ensured only by keeping the patient in hospital, arrangements should be made for staff from the service who know the dying person well to provide 24 hour cover if possible. This would enable staff to serve as a channel of communication between the patient and health care professionals and to provide advocacy on the patient's behalf.

Access to palliative care

It is very important that a patient should have access to palliative care services, which include nursing care, pain control and symptom management. Referral to these services is usually arranged by the patient's GP or district nurse. Palliative care can be provided within a hospice or hospital, within the patient's residential care environment or in their own home. It can take the form of nursing care or advice communicated to those undertaking the day to day nursing of the patient. If possible, individual care plans should be developed for each patient, and these may include pain relief, pressure care, physiotherapy, family support, the religious dimension and day services (Murdy and O'Leary, 1999). Day services can include Snoezelen sessions (time in a sensory room) and various therapeutic activities which are known to be enjoyed by the patient.

The Hospice Information Service publishes a directory listing all palliative care services throughout the United Kingdom and Republic of Ireland (see Useful Addresses).

Cancer care

For cancer patients, palliative care expertise can be provided through the NHS by Macmillan Cancer Relief and Marie Curie Cancer Care – both charitable bodies – (see Useful Addresses), by means of referral by the patient's GP or district nurse. The district nurse, who is contacted through the patient's GP, is responsible for assessing patients' nursing requirements.

Macmillan Nurses, who work in hospitals and in the community, advise on pain control and symptom management, give guidance on treatments available and offer psychological and emotional support to patients and carers.

Marie Curie Nurses give practical nursing care to patients throughout the day, overnight in their own homes or in the Marie Curie Centres, which offer a wide spectrum of palliative care expertise. The caring role is extended to a limited number of patients with life-shortening illnesses other than cancer. The practical role of Marie Curie Nurses complements that of the Macmillan Nurses, whose role is mainly advisory. In some cases patients benefit from both types of nursing simultaneously, depending upon their needs.

Issues relating to palliative care for people with learning disabilities

The integration of people with learning disabilities into the community has meant that most of them now depend on primary health care teams to meet their medical needs. Several studies have shown that the medical needs of many people with learning disabilities have been overlooked, thus delaying access to palliative care (Tuffrey-Wijne, 1997).

Various causes of this failure have been identified, including:
- communication impairment on the part of people with learning disabilities
- failure of carers to recognise symptoms of pain and illness
- mistaken attribution by health care staff of symptoms to the learning disability rather than the physical illness
- lack of health care screening generally available to the wider population.

Some suggested recommendations for overcoming this failure are:
- improved awareness by carers of signs and symptoms of early disease
- increased awareness of learning disability on the part of health care professionals
- improvement in health care screening (Tuffrey-Wijne, 1997).

A very important development in promoting access of people with learning disabilities to palliative care was the formation in November 1998 by The National Network for the Palliative Care of People with Learning Disabilities (see Useful Addresses). Among its aims are:
- to identify and promote good practice
- to provide information, training and research
- to highlight the need for ease of access for people with learning disabilities to mainstream palliative care services and the related need for the creation of some specialist learning disability care services.

Two groups of people with learning disabilities have been identified who are most in need of specialist palliative care services:
- those with profound disabilities who are unable to use verbal communication
- those with challenging behaviour.

(Murdy and O'Leary, 1999)

The Northgate and Prudhoe NHS Trust (see Useful Addresses) piloted a specialist in-patient service for these two groups of people as part of its aim of developing a specialist approach to palliative care. Unfortunately, the scheme closed due to financial constraints after referrals to the service did not reflect the perceived high level of need, although the specialist expertise of the staff involved has been valued by colleagues in mainstream services and learning disability services for clients who have palliative care needs (Murdy and O'Leary, 1999).

Relevance to people with autism

Issues relating to palliative care for people with learning disabilities are relevant to people with autism. The spectrum includes a significant number of people who fall into the two groups for whom mainstream palliative care services are not considered appropriate – those with a severe communication disorder and those with challenging behaviour. They would therefore need specialist palliative care services, whether in a hospice, hospital or their own living environment.

However, the needs of many people with autism are so complex that even if they do not fall within the two groups mentioned above, specialised palliative care services might have to be devised for them on the initiative of the staff who normally serve as their carers, working in co-operation with specialist nurses.

Commitment to the dying

It is hoped that among the staff who have demonstrated a strong commitment to ensuring the best possible quality of life to each person with autism in their care, there will always be available some who, when called upon to do so, will demonstrate an equally strong commitment to ensuring them a fearless and peaceful death.

APPENDICES

Grief reactions of people with autistic spectrum disorders

Appendix I was compiled from the results of a survey undertaken for the paper on *The management of bereavement in services for people with autism*, published in 1992. A total of 20 respondents to a notice in *Communication* (The National Autistic Society members' magazine), among whom were both parents and care staff, completed a questionnaire on individuals with autism whom they had supported during their grieving process. Ten responses which were considered to represent the breadth of the spectrum are included in this appendix. It is likely that several of them would now be diagnosed as having Asperger syndrome. One of the two additional contributions received from parents who did not complete the questionnaire referred to their family member as having Asperger syndrome.

Appendix II resulted from a request for those who supported people with Asperger syndrome through the grieving process. Only two responses were received, one from parents and one from care staff. In addition, a young man with Asperger syndrome offered a very moving account of his bereavement experience.

Those concerned with the management of bereavement in services for people with autism have reason to be grateful to those who participated in the two surveys. A particular debt of gratitude is owed to the relatives who helped with this study, and to the young man with Asperger syndrome, as in so doing they were reliving their own experiences of bereavement.

All of the contributions have been valuable, both in providing background for the book and in validating its recommendations. They demonstrate how sensitive management can help bereaved people with autistic spectrum disorders towards a successful resolution of grief.

The names of the bereaved have been changed in order to preserve confidentiality.

APPENDIX I

Grief reactions of people with autism

Alan

Age at time of bereavement: 14

Description
Highly dependent, needing constant supervision and frequent physical intervention. Able to converse and express preferences and feelings; some ritualistic behaviour; a high level of anxiety; hyperactive; mood swings; epileptic.
- In residential school: termly boarding at time of bereavement.

Relationship to deceased
Grandmother. Close and affectionate.

How was bereaved told of death?
Mother told him, 'Nana was very ill, so Jesus invited her to his wonderful garden. She is happy now and wants you to know she will always love you.'

Immediate reactions
Ran round the room with grief. Then cuddled by his mother and cried on her shoulder. He said, 'Mummy, I do love you,' then, 'Nana, oh my Nana.' Shock then set in and he did not speak for three days.

Later reactions
Epileptic attacks; temperature; lethargy; depression; disinterested in food and drink; stomach upset. He said he was sad and frightened and was unresponsive. Concerned about mother's health. Tried to hurry past end of road where grandmother lived and did not wish to visit her house again.

Funeral and rituals
Did not attend funeral. Took flowers to the crematorium garden, but refused to visit ever again. Will not look towards it when he passes.

Support
Warm support from mother. Assurance that Nana did not 'go away' and that he could talk about his sadness. Demonstrations of caring and affection (physical contact).

Resolution of grief
Happy to have his grandmother's radio, a clock and some of her pictures. Speaks of her often, for example, 'Nana liked those autumn tints,' 'Is Nana pleased with me?'

Derek

Age at time of bereavement: 17

Description
Dependent and needing constant supervision in living and working. Speech very limited but can express preferences and feelings. Usually cheerful but sometimes sad or worried. Occasional challenging behaviour when feeling insecure. Some periods of anxiety.
- Termly boarder at school at time of bereavement.

Relationship to deceased
Father. Close and affectionate.

How was bereaved told of death?
His mother told him, 'Daddy is in heaven.'

Type of death
Death was anticipated but bereaved did not know of illness.

Immediate reactions
Disbelief. He asked, 'Where is Daddy?' and was told, 'In heaven.' Afterwards he did not comment.

Later reactions
No indication of awareness of loss. Asked again, 'Where is Daddy?'

Funeral and rituals
Did not participate in any bereavement rituals.

Support
Staff at school and his mother who arranged for the bereaved to have frequent home visits and who ensured that he was aware of her affection for him.

Resolution of grief
Difficult to detect as no apparent grieving process.

Subsequent bereavements

Grandfather died five years later. He was told, 'Grandad is in heaven', and appeared undisturbed. He never asked about him again. The family dog died nine years after his father. The bereaved was told, 'Kelly is in heaven with Daddy and Grandad.' He continues to speak of him as though he were alive, i.e. 'Take Kelly for a walk.'

Comments

Mother is concerned about the effect of her own death on her son and is pleased that her sister and elder son make a practice of arranging for him to visit them, particularly when she is on holiday.

Donald

Age at time of bereavement: 29

Description
Dependent and needing constant supervision in living and working. Very articulate. Normally stable, but anxiety caused by unexpected events, and challenging behaviour only when disturbed. Very much concerned about world events e.g. nuclear threat, world ecology.
- Living at home and a day patient at an industrial therapy unit at the time of bereavement.

Relationship to deceased
Brother. Close and affectionate.

How was bereaved told of death?
At the time of death he was on holiday at a Steiner community familiar to him because he had frequently spent periods of time there. As he had attended Steiner schools before, he accepted their religious beliefs, including a firm belief in an after-life. Death was explained in these terms.

Type of death
Death was sudden.

Immediate reactions
No particular changes in behaviour but a great need to talk about the deceased and the effect of the loss on his own life as deceased really cared about him. Read his obituaries, looked at photographs, looked at slides the deceased had sent him.

Funerals and rituals
Bereaved away from home and did not attend funeral.

Support
Staff well known to him helped him through the first few weeks with excellent counselling. He was able to speak about his loss.

Later reactions
Talks about death frequently. He has signed a consent form for his brain to be used

Appendix I

for research after death. Anticipates that parents (in their seventies) will die soon. It is predicted that when his mother dies his behaviour will become very disturbed, if not violent. He realises that her death could mean loss of the family home. Talks of committing suicide when both parents are dead (previously, when depressed, made an attempt). Hopes he will not live to old age.

Religious beliefs

Greatly influenced by Steiner philosophy. Firm belief in an after-life in which he will have no disability and in which he will be able to do all the things he has not been able to do in this life.

Comments

For ten years the anniversary of his brother's death was marked by rituals of reading his obituaries, looking at photographs and at slides sent to him by the deceased. On the tenth anniversary, he said this would be the last one to be marked by the usual ceremonies and that he could not go on mourning forever.

Dorothy

Age at time of bereavement: 37

Description
Dependent but requiring supervision in living and working and, with occasional physical intervention, able to express preferences and to converse. Occasional speech, occasional anxiety, ritualistic and obsessive when distressed, passive, equable with occasional anger, unable to express feelings.
- In residential care at time of bereavement.

Relationship to deceased
Father. Close and affectionate. Home visits (one or two weeks) four times a year. Postal contact every fortnight.

How was bereaved told of death?
Two members of staff. The one responsible for bereavement support spoke and the other was unobtrusively present to observe reactions. Death was explained in the same terms as that of her mother, who had died three years previously. She was told, 'Daddy's pain has stopped, he has died and is in heaven with Mummy. The cat is being cared for by neighbours.'

Type of death
The bereaved knew that her father was ill. She had not gone home for the summer holiday.

Immediate reactions
Client apparently understood the loss immediately. She said 'Daddy.' She went very quiet and was later heard talking in the accent she uses when re-living early memories.

Later reactions
Subdued for several days. On being questioned by another resident about her forthcoming holiday she said, 'I am not going home because Daddy has gone to heaven,' without appearing upset. Showed signs of impatience when things could not be done immediately and less talkative with staff. General irritability.

Funerals and rituals

Attended funeral accompanied by two staff members. She did not join in with the singing as she would normally, but no other unusual reactions. Present at cremation and committal. The service meant very little to her and she did not ask about the coffin. She visited the family home and very much enjoyed talking with relatives and guests. Her brother sorted out records and mementoes for her to keep. On leaving she said, 'Dad wasn't home today.' She seemed to accept the reminder that Daddy was in heaven with Mummy. On the way home she was heard to say, 'When Dad's back from heaven, I will go home on the coach.'

Support

Mature staff member who accompanied her to the funeral and was regularly available and on-call if not on-duty.

Long-term reactions

Questionnaire completed before these could be determined. It is believed that the previous bereavement had given the client some understanding of death. It has been observed that she interacts more with staff and other clients than she did before her bereavement.

Elizabeth

Age at time of bereavement: 20

Description
Dependent and needing supervision in living and working. Communicates with ease and able to converse; suffers episodes of anxiety which can be resolved if reason is known; frequently obsessive and ritualistic; pinches herself; challenging behaviour in response to certain words, objects, music and also the death of her brother; very high mathematical ability - 'savant', and also artistic.
• In residential care at time of bereavement.

Relationship to deceased
Brother. Close and affectionate.

How was bereaved told of death?
Stepmother explained that her brother had been taken up to heaven because he had been 'poorly' and also had a sore leg. He was no longer in pain and was happy now.

Immediate reactions
She wanted to know when it happened and at what time. She was angry because her brother had left her.

Later reactions
It was one week before she cried and realised she would not see her brother again. When contact with him would normally have occurred – she had gone home every weekend and holidays – she became depressed, aggressive, tore clothes and self-harmed. Her sleeping pattern changed and she became destructive. She was prescribed medication for severe depression. Also complained of headaches, stomach pains and a very sad feeling in her heart, and fears of her own death. Suffered a nightmare centred on her brother, a 'black hole in the ground' [grave]. Questions centred on the 'black hole in the ground.' She dreamed that her father was forcing her to eat meat which was her brother's flesh. She asked questions about heaven and spoke of hearse, coffin and graves.

Funeral and rituals
The family considered it unwise for her to attend.

Support
Senior care worker who was available to counsel, listen and comfort and who talked to her, explaining that heaven was a wonderful place. She asked her to look at the sky and see how peaceful it looked and told her it was good to cry. She took her to church to light candles on her brother's birthday and 'talk' to him.

Comments
Bereaved has been able to offer reassurance to a client whose grandmother died and also to a bereaved member of staff.

Frederick

Age at time of bereavement: 20

Description
Moderately able and can live and work with partial autonomy. Problems of motivation; able to converse; ritualistic in small things; anxious if routine is disturbed; verbal abuse if anxiety is acute; otherwise, equable and passive.
- Living at home and holding an independent job in the community at time of bereavement.

Relationship to deceased
Father. Emotionally distant.

Previous bereavement
Lost grandfather whom he loved. Spoke about him, for example, 'Would Grandad have been at the cricket match?'

How was bereaved told of death?
Mother said, 'Daddy had a heart attack and the doctors could not help him to get well, so God took him to heaven to make him better.'

Type of death
Death was sudden.

Immediate reactions
No emotion. He put soup spoon down and said, 'Are you all right, Mum?' 'Why can't Charles [foster brother] come home and be head of this family?' 'I don't want a stepfather.' Understood loss immediately and reacted by fulfilling father's tasks such as coal carrying, walking the dog and cleaning the car.

Later reactions
Followed normal routines. Watched father's cricket team as usual, sitting at tea with the cricketers as though father was still present. Blinked back tears when looking at father's photograph. Accepted mother changing her seat at the table (taking father's chair). This was surprising as he is normally fiercely resistant to change. Took mother's hand when going to church a week after father's death when normally he would not have walked with her. Became more responsive to mother,

Appendix I

helping with household tasks not previously undertaken, such as cutting the grass. Did not express grief verbally. After one year took a keen interest in mother's male friends, expressing regret if relationship broke down.

Funeral and rituals
Present at funeral and cremation. Smiled at congregation as he passed them.

Support
A close male friend of his mother and father took over some of father's caring role such as taking him to football matches and buying him an electric razor.

Resolution of grief
Mother has tried to encourage him to speak of father but without success. He continually looks at family photographs, including those of early childhood. Has totally accepted his step-father. He tells him, 'I will call you Dad when you marry Mum.'

Comments
Duration of grieving process two years. Support of father's friend in ensuring continuity of normal activities.

Harriet

Age at time of bereavement: 34

Description
Dependent and requiring supervision in living and working. Very limited language but able to express preferences; able to express thoughts and feelings in writing, but only with mother; high level of anxiety and many fears (death, wars, natural disasters, accidents to parents). Usually reassurance and diversion can ensure she is settled and happy, but occasionally nothing can alleviate her anxiety, in which case challenging and compulsive behaviour can result.
- In residential care at time of bereavement.

Relationship to deceased
Grandfather. Close and affectionate. Saw him most days when she lived at home. After she went to residential care, he stayed at the family home during her visits.

How was bereaved told of death?
Key worker told her that Grandpa had died peacefully: he was not ill but very old. Three months before the death, her mother had broken her hip when Harriet was on a home visit. On return to residential care she lost weight and exhibited challenging behaviour. Staff and her parents agreed to delay telling her of grandfather's death until after she had seen her mother walking normally again and her behaviour had settled.

Type of death
Death was anticipated. She appeared to realise that her grandfather was failing well before he died. He was unable to visit the family home during one holiday and on her return staff noticed disturbed behaviour. Staff believed this resulted from a change in medication but her parents were convinced it was her awareness of impending loss.

Immediate reaction
Accepted news calmly.

Later reaction
When parents visited, they noticed she had scratches on her hands and face. There were tears when grandfather was mentioned and she appeared grief-stricken. Later

Appendix I

she wrote, 'We are sad to think of Grandpa in his coffin.' Many times she said that he was in his house and would come back.

Funeral and rituals
Because of distance and necessary delay in telling client of the death, she did not attend the funeral.

Support
Very caring key worker who gave her extra attention. She shrank from physical contact.

Previous bereavements
Grandmother died 13 years previously and client reacted with some disturbance. Two other deaths known to her. All deaths increase her anxiety about her own parents' deaths.

Resolution of grief
Later she wrote that she knew the happy times with Grandpa would not return but that she remembered them.

Duration of grieving process
Six months before death and six months after it.

Religious beliefs
Influenced by attendance at Steiner School and Christian beliefs. Parents have explained that we meet our loved ones in the after-life.

Larry

Age at time of bereavement: 3
(age when questionnaire completed: 20)

Description
Highly dependent and needing constant supervision and frequent physical intervention. Able to speak with difficulty; bangs his head to force words out (not yet able to speak at time of bereavement). Panic attacks; obsessive; collecting objects which others would discard; self-harm.

Relationship to deceased
Grandfather. Close and affectionate. Lived in the same house.

How was bereaved told of death?
Mother said, 'Grandad has died and is not in pain anymore.'

Type of death
Death was anticipated. Larry was aware that his grandfather was in hospital during the fortnight before his death.

Immediate reactions
Screamed on the evening of funeral. Not long after funeral he was humming parts of Beethoven's Ninth Symphony, one of his grandfather's favourites.

Later reactions
Screaming at bed-time – his grandfather used to play violin and sing to him at bed-time; humming Beethoven; appeared to be in pain; prone to infections, anxiety and hyperactivity.

Funerals and rituals
Not present at funeral but was taken to the burial by a neighbour. On later occasions helped to tidy the grave and waved good-bye.

Resolution of grief
Bereaved used to speak of 'Grandad at the cemetery,' but now no longer mentions him.

Appendix I

Anniversary of death
Anxiety around the time of the anniversary of death, but this was also the date of Larry's first visit to the hospital residence where he now resides.

Long-term reactions
Wanting to die/afraid of dying.

Comments
Mother describes Larry's life as a series of bereavements: losing his grandfather at the age of three; sent by Local Authority to weekly boarding school 25 miles from his home at age seven; losing father through failure of parents' marriage; admitted to permanent residence in hospital at age 12. He is not allowed to visit home as staff say that he is 'too attached' to it, nor is his grandmother, of whom he is fond, allowed to visit him. He cannot listen to Beethoven's Ninth Symphony as it makes him feel 'too sad.'

Malcolm

Age at time of bereavement: 28 (father), 31 (mother)

Description
Moderately able and can live and work with partial autonomy. Extremely chatty; high and frequent anxiety; obsessional, especially about antiques and china; relates well to elderly females; occasionally depressed, but changeable moods; passive, tendency to laziness.
- In residential care at the time of bereavement.

Relationship to deceased
Ambivalent towards father; close and affectionate with mother.

Type of death
In both cases the bereaved knew they were ill.

Immediate reactions when told of deaths
Disbelief with father, anxious about him not really being dead, saying, 'Promise me he is really dead.' Soon afterwards he sought reassurance about his mother's health. When told of his mother's death, he said, 'Oh really?' It took two or three days for him to realise that he had suffered a loss. He then said, 'I miss her.'

Later reactions
Could talk about his father's death. Of his mother he said, 'I miss her.' After her death he became very dependent on staff. There was a marked increase in anxiety with related hyper-ventilation. He frequently expressed a sense of loss, particularly about home visits and being spoiled by his mother. He became very withdrawn on the first Mother's Day after his mother's death when he realised there was no point in sending a card.

Funeral and rituals
Understood significance of rituals. Father's funeral was a 'social event' for the bereaved where he exhibited no sense of loss. He attended mother's funeral, bought flowers and laid them on the coffin. He was very involved and expressed sadness at each stage, though he did not weep. He was able to share his feelings with other, older relatives.

Support
Mother after father's death and principal of residential service after mother's death. Encouraged to talk about the deceased; efforts made to ensure that staff were available to offer support.

Resolution of grief
Adjusted to loss of his father in less than a year. As the questionnaire was completed soon after the death of his mother, it is difficult to reach conclusions about resolution of grief. He still says, 'I miss her' and 'I haven't anywhere to go now.'

Matthew

Age at time of bereavement: 31

Description
Moderately able and capable of partial autonomous living and working. He is able to express feelings and converse easily, but rarely initiates conversation. He will always try to steer conversations in the direction of his own interests, e.g. to past personalities in his own life or 1960/70's celebrities. Suffers from anxiety deriving from overhearing conversations which he assumes are about himself. Exhibits rare challenging behaviour directed at his mother or people who remind him of her. Lack of confidence, cheerful at times, moody at others.
* In residential care at the time of bereavement.

Relationship to deceased
Father. Ambivalent.

How was the bereaved told of death?
Client cannot remember and relevant staff member has departed.

Immediate reactions
Very matter of fact.

Later reactions
Affects of bereavement unclear to staff. Bereaved is very matter of fact, referring to the deceased as 'my late father who's dead now.'

Funeral and ritual
Bereaved did not attend funeral on grounds that it would be too difficult for his mother. At the express request of his mother, the bereaved has not been permitted to visit the memorial stone. The client has acquiesced, not wishing to upset his mother.

Resolution of grief
No reference is made to the deceased by client. If someone else initiates the subject, he refers to the deceased as 'my late father who's dead now.'

Appendix I

Additional Contributions

(Illustrations of 'inappropriate reactions')

Bereaved: 13 year old boy (Asperger syndrome)

Parents were separated but the father maintained close contact with the boy. The father died suddenly and the boy returned to school on the following Monday, telling staff that 'two sad things had happened' the previous Saturday: his father had died and Crystal Palace had lost their football match. Since then he has spoken about his father's death in a very matter of fact way, with no apparent awareness of any emotional implications.

Bereaved: 16 year old girl (autistic with severe epilepsy)

When the bereavement occurred she was living in residential school. Her father died suddenly and her mother came to the school to inform her. She replied 'That's nice that daddy's gone to heaven.' Later, when shopping with her mother, she said, 'Oh, that's sad. You won't have to buy daddy's tea now.'

APPENDIX II

Grief reactions of people with Asperger syndrome

Alfred

Age at time of bereavement: 24

Description
Low independence skills; prone to high anxiety; very moody; social interactions are active but odd.
- In residential care, visiting home every third weekend.

Relationship to deceased
Grandmother. Close and affectionate.

How was bereaved told of death?
Parents explained, 'Nanny has died.'

Type of death
Death was sudden.

Immediate reactions
Quiet but calm.

Later reactions
He had many upsets at the residential home, but was deemed to be depressed and put on medication. The parents believed that he was exhibiting a normal grief reaction and that medication was ill-advised. Parents behaved very naturally with him, speaking of his grandmother frequently and recalling the good times they had together. They lit candles in churches with him.

Funeral and rituals
Attended cremation but didn't really understand how to react. He was very supportive to his cousins who were visibly upset.

Support
Lighting candles in memory of the deceased, talking with parents, extended family and staff.

Previous bereavement
Close family friend, aunt, grandfather, grandmother, uncle, teacher.

Resolution of grief
About 9-12 months, but when anxious will refer to all the people close to him who have died.

Alice

Age at time of bereavement: not given, but in a service for adults.

Description
Fearful that her new placement might not be permanent; anxious; suffering from low self-esteem; history of anorexia and bulimia (her deceased friend had also suffered from anorexia).
- At the time of bereavement in a residential service for people with Asperger syndrome to which she had recently been transferred.

Relationship to deceased
Female friend who was a resident in the service from which Alice had recently transferred.

How was bereaved told of death?
Staff told of the death.

Type of death
Death was by suicide.

Immediate reactions
She was told of the death on the same day she had a review of her new placement. The staff were unable to tell whether the anxiety she exhibited arose from her fear that her new placement might not be permanent or from the news of her friend's death.

Later reaction
A few weeks after hearing of her friend's death, she heard on the news that a fireman had been killed in the course of his duties and exhibited acute grief reactions. She showed more signs of grief over this man than at any time after her friend's death. She is obsessed with firemen and the fire service.

Support
The staff of the Service caring for her. They were aware that she might need support on the anniversary of her friend's death or the date of her friend's birthday.

Appendix II

George

Age at time of report: 31
(had recently been diagnosed as having Asperger syndrome)

In response to his request, he was sent the paper on 'The management of bereavement in services for people with autism' (1992). He then wrote a letter, from which the following are extracts.

'I had never thought about [bereavement]. Even though I have been to a few funerals, nothing ever stirred in me. I was just following everyone else and mimicking them. When I read through [the paper] I went into a state of shock. I was angry and confused... Then slowly I started to have... insights into some feelings and thoughts I have been trying to work out for years.

'I was overwhelmed with guilt and have been for a long time, 17 years at least. I [realised that] I had felt guilt because of my dog's death.

'When I was about 13-14 years, old my dog was old and dying... I was playing by myself as usual when I put my leg through a piece of glass. Suddenly my dog bit me and pulled me over. I kicked out and shouted at him. This is what I have felt guilty about. (Shortly afterwards the dog was put down).

'My dog was the only friend I ever had... I constantly got things wrong and was punished by my parents. I was safe with him, sitting next to him and feeling his soft brown coat. I think my dog was my only real source of giving and receiving love. I have cried about my dog as visions of him have entered my mind. I am beginning to realise that my family interaction was and still is distant. I am realising that I had some sort of love for my dog, a love which I find hard to understand with other people

'My dog died when I was 13 years of age. At the time I felt nothing. I was told he had gone but this had no meaning for me. This is the time I started to feel bad about my behaviour and a self-consciousness was forming, but all I knew is that I was told I was bad and so thought I was bad.

'When I was 21 years of age my favourite auntie died. This was the first funeral ritual that I attended. I was just following and mimicking everyone else. I never really understood why people were crying and I didn't express any emotion... A year later another auntie died. I attended this funeral but again nothing stirred in me. When I was 27 years of age my mother's boyfriend died. Again I went to the funeral and acted out the emotions of others.

There were a number of other bereavements, starting from when he was four years of age, when he was left in the back of a car on his own during his grandmother's funeral. Later ones included the death of his grandfather, a friend from nursery school and an uncle (not known about at the time) and the death of a pet mouse.

'Out of all these issues of bereavement, I have trouble feeling or responding to them, expect for one, my dog Ringo... This is the only one that means anything to me and the only one where I can express real tears and emotion. One of the problems I have with emotions and feelings is that this concept is new to me, for it is only in the last four years that I have understood that this concept exists and is natural. I am still trying to understand feelings and how they interact with the rest of me. Self-awareness is something I have to learn about... Even though in my mind I know that people die, this means nothing to me. I suppose the semantic pragmatics of death and the difficulty I have in understanding this is like my problem with understanding interpersonal relationships and concepts like that of God.

'But what is confusing is this feeling of guilt that I have identified with my dog, for it is the same feeling that in reflection I was made to feel by my parents and the schools because of how I behaved... It is the feeling that controlled me and my 'bad' behaviour. It's the feeling that triggered my intelligence to mimic and pretend to interact, even though I never knew why.

'The only extrapolation I can make is an intellectual one, where I have learnt that society and religion use the process of guilt as a form of control and that, perhaps due to my dog's death, I have become sensitive to guilt and this extremely heightened feeling inside of me. A lot of pain and confusion has come from this because I didn't understand what was happening inside of me... I shall have to work to be able to understand and articulate. In time I will achieve this, but for the moment I am riding my bicycle without a chain.'

About nine months after writing this letter, he wrote another on the occasion of the death of his younger sister, from which the following are extracts:

Appendix II

'This has been a very challenging time and an opportunity for me to practise the issues of bereavement I learned with you last year. I was able to help the rest of my family though the range of emotions associated with grief as I had learnt them. I took an active role in helping to organise the funeral as my family were upset. People often said 'I was coping very well', but they don't understand that emotionally I am at a distance and that it will only be in the future that I may suffer as I finally work the grief out.

But for the moment I am trying to do the right things. I visited my sister a few times while she was in the mortuary and when I hugged her I got upset because this was the only time I could do this. It upset me that I could hug an inanimate person but not when she was alive. I placed photos and a gold chain in the coffin so I could always remember this in future when my feelings finally understand what has happened. I also made some booklets for the funeral so that she would always be remembered. But for now all I can do is carry on with my life and try to be the best I can.

'Once again, thank you for making me aware about bereavement and helping me to do the right thing while I had the opportunity. Otherwise I would have done nothing and would probably have felt guilty

REFERENCES

Bereavement

Attwood, T. (1993) *Why does Chris do that?*. London: The National Autistic Society. Available from The National Autistic Society Publications, tel: 020 7903 3595.

Attwood, T. (1998) *Asperger's syndrome: a guide for parents and professionals.* London: Jessica Kingsley. Available from The National Autistic Society Publications, tel: 020 7903 3595.

Attwood, T. (1999) Personal correspondence with author.

Attwood, T. (2000) 'Strategies for improving the social integration of children with Asperger syndrome', *Autism* 4 (1): 85-100.

Benefits Agency (1999) *What to do after a death in England and Wales,* Leaflet D49.

Brelstaff, K. (1984) 'Reactions to death: can the mentally handicapped grieve? Some experiences of those who did', *Teaching and Training* 22(1): 10-16.

The Caring Programme leaflet: *Coping with grief:* The Washington Home, 3720 Upton Street, NW, Washington DC 20016, USA.

Carr, A.T. (1988) 'Dying and bereavement' in J. Hall (ed) *Psychology for nurses and health visitors*, Chap. 7. London: Macmillan.

Cathcart, F. (1994) (three booklets) *Understanding Death and Dying:* 1. *Your feelings,* 2. *A guide for family and friends* 3. *A guide for carers and other professionals.* Kidderminster: British Institute for Learning Disabilities.

Day, K. (1985) 'Psychiatric disorder in the middle-aged and elderly mentally handicapped', *British Journal of Psychiatry* 147: 660-667.

Emerson, P. (1977) 'Covert grief reactions in mentally retarded clients', *Mental Retardation*, 15(6): 46-47.

Gerland, G. (1999) Letter to the Editor: 'Autism and psychodynamic theories', *Autism* 3 (3): 309-311.

Gillberg, C. (1991) 'Clinical and neurobiological aspects of Asperger syndrome in six family studies', in U. Frith (ed) *Autism and Asperger syndrome*, pp. 122-146, chapter 4. Cambridge: Cambridge University Press.

Gray, C.A. (1998) 'Social stories and comic strip conversations with students with Asperger syndrome and high-functioning autism', in E. Schopler, G.B. Mesibov and L.J. Kunce (eds) *Asperger syndrome or high-functioning autism?* pp. 167-198. New York: Plenum.

Harris, P. (1998) *What to do when someone dies*. London: Which? Ltd.

Hayworth, M. (1996) 'Explaining death', in B. Ward and associates *Good grief* (2), pp. 34-36. London: Jessica Kingsley.

Hollins, S. and Sireling, L. (1994) *When Dad died*. London: St George's Mental Health Library.

Hollins, S. and Sireling, L. (1999) *Understanding grief; working with grief and people who have learning disabilities*. Brighton: Pavilion.

Jordan, R. and Powell, S. (1995) *Understanding and teaching children with autism*. Chichester: Wiley. Available from The National Autistic Society Publications Department, tel: 020 7903 3595.

Kane, B. (1979) 'Children's concepts of death', *Journal of Genetic Psychology* 134: 141-153.

Kitching, N. (1987) 'Helping people with mental handicaps cope with bereavement', *Mental Handicap* 15, June: 60-63.

McCormick, J. (1998) 'Growing up - tackling depression', in *The autistic spectrum – a handbook 1999*, pp. 64-69. London: The National Autistic Society.

McLoughlin, I.J. (1986) 'Bereavement in the mentally handicapped', *British Journal of Hospital Medicine* 36(4): 256-260.

Morgan, H. (1996) *Adults with autism: a guide to theory and practice.* Cambridge: Cambridge University Press.

The National Autistic Society (1997) *How many people have autistic spectrum disorders?* London: The National Autistic Society. Reprinted 2001. Available from The National Autistic Society Information Centre, tel: 020 7903 3599.

The National Autistic Society (1998) 'Questions and answers about autistic spectrum disorders', in *The autistic spectrum – a handbook* 1999, pp. 29-35. London: The National Autistic Society.

Oswin, M. (1991) *Am I allowed to cry? A study of bereavement amongst people who have learning difficulties.* London: Souvenir Press.

Parkes, C.M. (1996) *Bereavement, studies of grief in adult life.* London: Routledge.

Parkes, C.M., Laugani, P. and Young, B (eds.) (1997) *Death and bereavement across cultures.* London: Routledge.

Pincus, L. (1961) 'Understanding loss' in B. Ward and associates *Good grief* (2) (1996) pp. 17-19. London: Jessica Kingsley.

Prior, M. (2000) 'Editorial', *Autism* 4 (1) : 5-8.

Rawlings, D. (1996, unpublished.) '*Have I finished being sad?*'

Rawlings, D. (1998, unpublished.) '*An investigation into the effects of bereavement in adults with autism living in residential care services, and an examination of the implications for service providers.*'

Schaeffer, D. and Lyons, C. (1998) *How do we tell the children?* New York: Newmarket Press.

Sireling, L. 'Life after death' (unpublished. paper) quoted in Kitching, N (1987) 'Helping people with mental handicaps cope with bereavement', *Mental Handicap* 15, June : 60-63.

Staudacher, C. (1988) *Beyond grief, a guide for recovering from the death of a loved one*. London: Souvenir Press.

Stickney, D. (1984) *Water bugs and dragon flies*. London: Mowbray.

Tantam, D. (2000) 'Psychological disorder in adolescents and adults with Asperger syndrome', *Autism* 4 (1): 47-62.

Turner, M. (1998) *Talking with children and young people about death and dying, a workbook*. London: Jessica Kingsley.

Ward, B. et al (1996) *Good grief (2), exploring feelings, loss and death with over elevens and adults, a holistic approach*. London: Jessica Kingsley.

Wertheimer, A. (1991) *A special scar, the experiences of people bereaved by suicide*. London: Routledge.

Wolff, S. (1995) *Loners, the life path of unusual children*. London: Routledge.

Worden, J.W. (1991) *Grief counselling and grief therapy, a handbook for the mental health practitioner*. London: Routledge.

Yanok, J. and Beifus, J.A. (1993) 'Communicating about loss and mourning: death education for individuals with mental retardation', *Mental Retardation* 31(3): 144-147.

REFERENCES

Support for the dying

Dickenson, D. and Johnson, M. (eds) (1993) *Death, dying and bereavement*. London: Sage Publications.

Lansdown, R. (1996) 'Working with young people facing death', in B. Ward and associates *Good grief* (2), pp. 32-33. London: Jessica Kingsley.

Murdy, J. and O'Leary, L. (1999) 'Understanding the issues of palliative care for someone with a learning disability' in N. Blackman (ed) *Living with loss, helping people with learning disabilities to cope with bereavement and loss*, pp. 37-39. Brighton: Pavilion.

Parkes, C.M., Laugani, P. and Young, B. (eds.) (1997) *Death and bereavement across cultures*. London: Routledge.

Peberdy, A. (1993) 'Spiritual care of dying people', in Dickenson, D. and Johnson, M. (eds) *Death, dying and bereavement*, pp. 219-223. London: Sage Publications.

Read, S. (1998) 'The palliative care needs of people with learning disabilities', *International Journal of Palliative Nursing*, 4 (5): 246-251.

Tuffrey-Wijne, I. (1997) 'Palliative care and learning disabilities', *Nursing Times*, 93 (31), 30 July: 50-51.

USEFUL ADDRESSES

Bereavement

British Institute of Learning Disabilities (BILD)
Wolverhampton Road
Kidderminster
Worcestershire
DY10 3PP
Tel: 01562 850 251
Fax: 01562 851 970
Email: bild@bild.demon.co.uk
Website: www.bild.org.uk

BILD is committed to improving the quality of life for people with learning disabilities by advancing education and research and promoting ways of working with, and for, people with learning disabilities. It is a major provider of training and publisher of books and journals relating to learning disabilities.

The Compassionate Friends
53 North Street
Bristol
BS3 1EN
Helpline: 0117 953 9639
Tel: 0117 966 5202
Email: info@tcf.org.uk
Website: www.tcf.org.uk

A self-help organisation of bereaved parents offering friendship and understanding to other bereaved parents. The Bristol Office will put enquirers in touch with other parents in their area. (See Shadow of Suicide Group).

CRUSE Bereavement Care
CRUSE House
126 Sheen Road
Richmond
Surrey
TW9 1UR
Tel: 020 8940 4818 (local branches are listed in local telephone directories)

A national organisation offering help to all bereaved people through its national office and local branches. It offers individual counselling, social meetings and advice on practical matters relating to bereavement. Whenever possible, enquirers are directed to their local branch. If there is none, the Head Office has counsellors available to answer letters and talk on the telephone. They have a comprehensive list of books and leaflets which can be ordered from CRUSE House.

The National Autistic Society
393 City Road
London
EC1V 1NG
Tel: 020 7833 2299
Fax: 020 7833 9666
Helpline: 0870 600 8585
Information centre: 020 7903 3599
Email: nas@nas.org.uk
Website: www.nas.org.uk

The Society champions the rights and interests of people with autism and works to ensure that they and their families receive quality services appropriate to their needs. Amongst its activities are: managing schools and adult services, supporting local authorities in developing their own specialist services, publishing books and leaflets, organising conferences and training programmes, offering specialist diagnostic services and managing a helpline.

The Samaritans
The Upper Mill
Kingston Road
Ewell, Surrey
KT17 2AF
Tel: 020 8394 8300 (local branches are listed in local telephone directories)
Fax: 020 8394 8301
Helpline: 08457 909090
Email: jo@samaritans.org.uk
Website: www.samaritans.org.uk

A national service offering befriending to anyone feeling desperate, lonely, suicidal, or going through a personal crisis such as bereavement.

Shadow of Suicide Group (SCS)

A sub-group of The Compassionate Friends for parents of children who have taken their own lives. The SCS group can put parents in touch with others similarly bereaved.
Tel: 0117 953 9639 (same as The Compassionate Friends)

Humanist and non-religious funerals/cremations
British Humanist Association
47 Theobalds Road
London
WC1X 8SP
Tel: 020 7420 0908

National Secular Society
25 Red Lion Square
London
WC1R 4RL
Tel/Fax: 020 7404 3126

These organisations will enable contact with the nearest official. It is usual to pay a fee and transport expenses.

Support for the dying

Hospice Information Service
St. Christopher's Hospice
51-59 Lawrie Park Road
Sydenham
London
SE26 6DZ
Tel: 020 8778 9252
Fax: 020 8659 8680

The Service publishes an annually updated directory of hospice and palliative care services in the UK and Republic of Ireland, sent free of charge on receipt of a large envelope and three first class stamps. Membership of the Service costs £30 per annum for which one receives the directory, a periodic bulletin and *Choices*, a list of all the palliative care courses in the UK. The head office at St. Christopher's Hospice runs a library and an education programme.

Macmillan Cancer Relief
89 Albert Embankment
London
SE1 7UQ
Information Line: 0845 601 6161
Fax: 020 7840 7841
Email: information_line@macmillan.org.uk
Website: www.macmillan.org.uk

There are over 1,700 Macmillan Nurses working in hospitals and in the community throughout the UK. They help in the following ways:

- advice on pain control and symptom management
- advice and guidance to patients on the different treatments available
- offering psychological and emotional support to patients and carers
- identifying sources of practical help.

The service is available to NHS patients via referral by their GP or district nurse. Some Macmillan Nurses specialise in particular cancers.

The 200 Macmillan Doctors, ranging from consultants to GPs, are based either in hospitals or in the community. Macmillan funds an educational programme available to other doctors and nurses, and they work with the NHS to provide day and in-patient units, treatment and information centres.

Marie Curie Cancer Care
89 Albert Embankment
London
SE1 7TP
Tel: 020 7599 7777
Fax: 020 7599 7788
Email: info@mariecurie.org.uk
Website: www.mariecurie.org.uk

Thousands of Marie Curie Nurses across the UK give practical nursing care to people with cancer, throughout the day or night, in their own homes and free of charge. Referral to the service is by the patient's GP or district nurse.

Palliative care is provided in ten Marie Curie centres, which offer specialised care for in-patients and out-patients, day care and home visits. They offer symptom control, pain relief, physiotherapy, respite care and terminal care as well as emotional and spiritual support. The caring role is also extended to a limited number of patients with life-threatening illnesses other than cancer who can benefit from the charity's specialist palliative care expertise. Marie Curie Cancer Care provides the largest number of hospice beds outside the NHS.

Other activities are research at the Marie Curie Research Institute and the Education Service, which runs courses and training programmes on many aspects of cancer and palliative care.

The National Network for the Palliative Care of People with Learning Disabilities
Cancer Services, Room 6CC03
Charing Cross Hospital
Fulham Palace Road
London W6 8RF
Tel: 020 8846 1739 or 1629
Fax: 020 8383 0612

The Network has regional representatives in England and Scotland. Its aims include:

- to identify and promote good practice in palliative care of people with learning disabilities locally and nationally
- to serve as a resource of information, training and research on palliative care for people with learning disabilities
- to highlight the need for increased ease of access of people with learning disabilities to mainstream palliative care services and related need for creation of some specialist learning disability care services
- to offer opportunities for the 'cross-fertilisation' of specialist knowledge of those working in the field of learning disability and those in the field of palliative care.

Northgate and Prudhoe NHS Trust
Northgate Hospital
Morpeth
Northumberland
NE61 3BP
Contact: Unit Manager, Medical Centre
Tel: 01670 394 125
Fax: 01670 394 005

The hospital provides four dedicated palliative beds for people with learning disabilities with a palliative care approach team being responsible for patient care. It is hoped that a full palliative care service can be set up in the future with established funding and support and with the following aims:

- to provide a palliative care approach for people with learning disabilities for whom mainstream services are not appropriate
- to support relatives and carers of the patients
- to share advice and support with other palliative care professionals working with people with learning disabilities.

INDEX

A

able autistic people	24, 31, 37, 52, 61, 62
grief reactions	49-50, 89-94
therapeutic measures	43, 44, 47
absence of grief	48
accidental death	38
address, forms of	26
advocates *see* citizen advocates	
after life beliefs	37, 42
ageing parents	16
aggression	35, 55
see also challenging behaviour; self-injurious behaviour	
anger reactions	35, 45, 55
anniversaries	13, 53
annual review meetings	19, 22
anticipated death	34
anxiety	
about death	30-31
following bereavement	45-46, 60
Asperger syndrome *see* able autistic people	
autism, definition	11
autistic people	
absence of grief	48
communicating with	61-62
difficulties in bereavement	48-53
explaining death to	28-30, 38-39
grief reactions	12, 67, 69-94
informing about deaths	35-39, 56
personal characteristics	25, 42
preparation for bereavement	27-28
see also able autistic people	
autistic spectrum disorders, definition	11

B

befrienders	21, 25, 44
behaviour *see* aggression; challenging behaviour; self-injurious behaviour	
behaviour therapy see cognitive behaviour therapy	
beliefs, after life	37, 42
bereaved people, support	12, 15, 17-20, 21-22, 24, 26, 29, 31-32, 42-43, 62-64
bereavement	
anxiety following	45-46, 60
definition	12
difficulties of autistic people	48-53
informing other parties of	39
preparation	27-28
bereavement support groups	18, 24, 33-34, 55-56
bereavement support workers	33, 42-43, 56, 60-61
bodies, viewing	40-41
British Humanist Association	26, 103
British Institute of Learning Disabilities	31, 101
brothers *see* siblings	

C

cancer care	64
organisations	104, 105
care *see* palliative care; support	
ceremonies *see* funerals; memorial services	
challenging behaviour	50
see also aggression	
citizen advocates	20-22, 25, 44
clients *see* service users	
cognitive behaviour therapy	43, 46
comfort *see* palliative care; support, for bereaved people	
comic strip conversations *see* social stories	

communication
- with dying service users — 61-62
- impairment in — 42
- *see also* non-verbal communication; verbal communication

The Compassionate Friends — 18, 101
counselling — 43, 47, 51
CRUSE — 18, 23, 31, 32, 56, 57, 102
cultural background — 23, 26

D

death
- anticipated — 34
- anxiety about — 30-31
- arrangements following — 56
- distorted understanding of — 31
- explaining to autistic people — 28-30, 38-39
- informing about — 35-39, 56
- mode of — 14, 38-39
- preoccupation with unrelated — 52
- of service users — 22-24, 56
- spiritual aspects — 29-30
- sudden — 35, 53

denial — 62
departure, of staff — 28
depression — 38, 43, 46-47
diet — 62-63
disruptive behaviour — 50
doctors *see* health professionals
dying people, location for — 63
dying relatives, visiting — 34
dying service users, communication with — 61-62

E

ethnic background — 23, 26
exercise — 46, 50, 51

F

families	
involving	17
of service users	25-26, 28, 61
support for	55, 57
see also parents; relatives; siblings	
fear *see* anxiety	
financial settlements	19, 20, 22
forms of address	26
friends, of service users	61
funeral arrangements	19-20, 22, 23-24, 41
funerals	26, 92-93
future planning	17, 19-22

G

graves, visiting	41
grief	
absence of	48
process	13-14, 39-42
for autistic people	12, 48-53
reactions	
of able autistic people	49-50, 89-94
of autistic people	12, 67, 69-94
of learning disabled people	12
symptoms	13, 14, 44-45, 47, 89-90, 92-94
guilt	45, 92, 93, 94

H

health professionals	61, 63, 64
homicide	39
Hospice Information Service	59, 63, 104
humanist funerals	26

I

informing autistic people about deaths	35-39, 56
informing other parties of bereavement	39

K
key workers　　　　　　　　　　　　　　　　33, 60

L
learning disabled people
   grief reactions　　　　　　　　　　　　　12
   medical needs　　　　　　　　　　　　　64-65
   see also able autistic people; autistic people
life story books　　　　　　　　　　　　　　28
literal interpretations　　　　　　　　　　　37
location, for dying people　　　　　　　　　63
lone parents　　　　　　　　　　　　　　　 16
loss of skills　　　　　　　　　　　　　　　48
losses
   everyday　　　　　　　　　　　　　　　28
   previous　　　　　　　　　　　　　　　 15, 25

M
Macmillan Cancer Relief　　　　　　　　　64, 104
Marie Curie Cancer Care　　　　　　　　　64, 105
medical needs, of learning disabled people　64-65
medication　　　　　　　　　　　　　　　 44, 46, 47, 50
mementoes　　　　　　　　　　　　　　　 42
memorial services　　　　　　　　　　　　41-42, 57
memorial stones, visiting　　　　　　　　　41
memory books　　　　　　　　　　　　　　28
mode of death　　　　　　　　　　　　　　14, 38-39
murder *see* homicide

N
National Autistic Society　　　　　　　　　11, 19, 20, 22, 32, 102
National Network for the Palliative Care of People
   with Learning Disabilities　　　　　　　 65, 105
National Secular Society　　　　　　　　　26, 103
natural death　　　　　　　　　　　　　　 38
nightmares　　　　　　　　　　　　　　　 47-48
non-religious funerals　　　　　　　　　　26

Index

non-verbal communication	24, 42, 60
see also verbal communication	
Northgate and Prudhoe NHS Trust	65, 106
nurses	64

P

palliative care	59-66, 105
panic *see* anxiety	
parents	11
future planning	17, 19-22
support for	16
see also successor parents	
people with autism *see* autistic people	
people with learning disabilities	
see learning disabled people	
personal information, on service users	25-26
planning, for the future	17, 19-22
preoccupation with unrelated death	52
preparation, for bereavement	27-28
priests *see* religious leaders	
psychodynamic therapies	43

Q

questionnaires	18-19, 20, 22

R

rabbis *see* religious leaders	
racial background	23, 26
regression	48
reincarnation	37
relatives	21
visiting	34
see also families; siblings	
relaxation	46, 50, 51
religions	29
religious background	23, 26, 44, 62
religious leaders	23-24, 26, 56, 62

resources, for training 31-32
review meetings 19, 22
rituals
   participation in 39-42
   see also funerals; memorial services

S

St Christopher's Hospice 59
Samaritans 18, 103
self-injurious behaviour 50-51
   see also aggression
service staff
   death of 56
   support 55-56
   training 18, 24, 26, 27, 31-32, 59
service users 11, 17-18
   communication with 61-62
   death 22-24, 56
   families 25-26, 28, 61
   informing of deaths 35-39
   personal information 25-26
services, memorial 41-42, 57
settlements *see* financial settlements
Shadow of Suicide Group 103
siblings 21
   see also families; relatives
single parents 16
sisters *see* siblings
skills, loss of 48
sleep difficulties 47-48
social interaction, impairment in 42
social stories 24, 44, 50, 51
spiritual aspects, of death 29-30
staff *see* service staff
successor parents 20-22, 44, 46
sudden death 35, 53

suicide | 37, 38-39, 47, 57, 103
support
   for bereaved people | 12, 15, 17-20, 21-22, 24, 26, 29, 31-32, 42-43, 62-64
   for parents | 16
   for staff | 55-56
   for surviving family members | 55, 57
support groups, for bereaved people | 18, 24, 33-34, 55-56
support workers, for bereavement | 33, 42-43, 56, 60-61
surviving family members, support | 55, 57
symptoms, of grief | 13, 14, 44-45, 47, 89-90, 92-94

T

terminally ill relatives, visiting | 34
therapeutic measures | 43, 46, 47, 50, 51, 63
training *see* service staff, training
training resources | 31-32
triad of impairments | 11

V

verbal communication | 24, 42, 60
   see also non-verbal communication
vicars *see* religious leaders
videos | 28
viewing, bodies | 40-41
visiting
   dying relatives | 34
   memorial stones | 41

W

wills | 19, 20, 22
Worden, J. W. | 14

Notes

Notes